MAJORING IN NURSING

From Prerequisites to
Postgraduate Study and Beyond

JANET R. KATZ,
RN, MSN, RN,C

Farrar, Straus and Giroux
New York

Farrar, Straus and Giroux
19 Union Square West, New York 10003

Copyright Q 1999 by Janet R. Katz
All rights reserved
Distributed in Canada by Douglas & McIntyre Ltd.
Printed in the United States of America
Designed by Peter Buchanan-Smith
First edition, 1999

5 7 9 10 8 6

Library of Congress Cataloging-in-Publication Data
Katz, Janet R., 1953–
    Majoring in nursing : from prerequisites to post graduate study
and beyond / Janet R. Katz. — 1st ed.
        p.   cm.
    ISBN 0-374-52567-6 (alk. paper)
    1. Nursing—Vocational guidance. I. Title.
RT82.K35   1999
610.73'06'09—dc21   98-15168

"Code for Nurses" on page xi is reprinted with permission
from *Code for Nurses with Interpretive Statements*, Q 1985, American Nurses
Publishing, American Nurses Foundation / American Nurses Association,
600 Maryland Avenue, SW, Suite 100W, Washington, DC 20024-2571.

The chart on page 83 is reprinted with permission of the
American Association of Colleges of Nursing.

To William Katz, the elder and the younger

ACKNOWLEDGMENTS

Thank you . . .

Kelly Fox, RN, BSN; Carol Carter, series editor; and Denise Oswald, editor and wielder of the green pencil. Martha Herman, Randy Katz, Chris Pozerycki, William Vincer Katz, Bill Katz, and Linda Sternberg Katz.

To all the nurses I interviewed for letting me use your wonderful stories in this book. To RNs around the world who do the work of caring even when it seems like nobody cares about you: stand up and make your voices heard for the health of people and the environment.

And to Gregg Godsey, who literally made writing a book possible.

CONTENTS

CODE FOR NURSES

1. The nurse provides services with respect for human dignity and the uniqueness of the client unrestricted by considerations of social or economic status, personal attributes, or the nature of health problems.

2. The nurse safeguards the client's right to privacy by judiciously protecting information of a confidential nature.

3. The nurse acts to safeguard the client and the public when health care and safety are affected by the incompetent, unethical, or illegal practice of any person.

4. The nurse assumes responsibility and accountability for individual nursing judgments and actions.

5. The nurse maintains competence in nursing.

6. The nurse exercises informed judgment and uses individual competence and qualifications as criteria in seeking consultation, accepting responsibilities, and delegating nursing activities to others.

7. The nurse participates in activities that contribute to the ongoing development of the profession's body of knowledge.

8. The nurse participates in the profession's efforts to implement and improve standards of nursing.

9. The nurse participates in the profession's efforts to establish and maintain conditions of employment conducive to high-quality nursing care.

10. The nurse participates in the profession's effort to protect the public from misinformation and misrepresentation and to maintain the integrity of nursing.

11. The nurse collaborates with members of the health professions and other citizens in promoting community and national efforts to meet the health needs of the public.

MAJORING IN NURSING

You Don't Have to Like Blood to Be a Nurse

I'm a registered nurse. Often when I tell someone this they say, "Oh, I could never be a nurse. I hate blood." Well, guess what? So do I. Nursing is about so much more than blood and it is the "much more" that I'll be telling you about in this book. You probably have an idea of what a nurse is, and unless you have a family member or close friend who not only is a nurse but talks about being a nurse, I think your idea is probably incomplete. This book will help you get a realistic picture of what being a registered nurse is all about.

There are good things and bad things about being a nurse, and as with all decisions, you need to weigh the pros and the cons. I suggest you keep a running list as you read this book. Make two columns and write Pros at the head of one, and Cons at the head of the other. These pros and cons are personal, they belong to you, so it doesn't matter what other people, like school counselors, family, or friends, think. When I write about how nurses need excellent communication skills and you're thinking about how you don't really like to talk to people, include that in your con list. If you wish to be less black-and-white about it, make your list with three or four columns marked Super Pro, Pro, Con, and Super Con. That way you can rate the degree, or weight, of each item.

Be honest with yourself; not everyone is going to make a great nurse, but at least give yourself the time to consider this rewarding and versatile career.

What Is a Nurse?

There are as many answers to that question as there are nurses, because nursing covers a lot of ground. Nurses work in so many different circumstances doing so many different things that it is hard to say that any one, two, or three things define what a nurse does. And this is exactly what makes nursing such an exciting profession. Nursing is filled with moments that are profoundly meaningful and at the same time difficult to measure or describe. How do you talk about the healing power of holding a hand? Or about an emergency department nurse who thinks it takes more skill to talk with a rape victim than to save the life of a trauma victim? How can nurses talk about saving lives when the doctor walks in, either in real life or on television, and gets all the credit?

Thus, it is not easy to tell someone what a nurse is, but the World Health Assembly in Geneva has done a fantastic job of answering that question. They recently called nurses "indispensable" contributors to worldwide national health programs and, further, praised nurses for their cost-effective high standards of providing quality care. Nurses were referred to as the "backbone" and the "heart" of health care who cross all geographic and political boundaries. To be internationally recognized in this way makes me proud to be a nurse.

A nursing degree can be used to work in or out of hospitals, in helicopters, on boats, and in the home. Nurses work for the United States government in the military, at the National Institutes of Health, at the Centers for Disease Control, and in Congress as representatives or senators. Nurses work internationally for relief organizations, large corporations, foreign schools, or small village clinics.

Nurses save lives, take care of people who are dying, provide pain relief, do scientific research, run hospitals, and design computer systems. With advanced degrees nurses deliver babies, run their own clinics, provide primary care, give anesthesia to people undergoing surgery, and become lawyers in medical law. All nurses are teachers and counselors and, in one way or another, help people live healthier lives.

I have three jobs right now: one is working in a cardiac rehabilitation center where I teach people with heart disease about exercise and lifestyle changes, the second is at a university teaching nursing students, and the third is writing for nursing publications. I love the flexibility, and as I've been writing this book, I've realized that I am doing exactly what I've always wanted to do—I'm not tied down to a nine-to-five office job. Mostly I work at home and still I have plenty of time through teaching and exercise classes to be with other people. I am continually learning new information, be it about health care economics, the pathophysiology of heart failure, or the psychological impact that the diagnosis of heart disease has on a thirty-eight-year-old. I love knowing that I could quit any of these jobs and find others. But what I especially love and cherish is how much I have grown as a person since becoming a nurse. I've learned more about what it means to be human than anything else, and I am grateful to the many different people I've learned this from.

I've been a nurse for fifteen years and, just so you know, I haven't always been so enthusiastic about nursing. Being a nurse is hard; there have been times when I wanted nothing more than to get out of nursing. Along the way I had to take a good hard look at what I was doing and ask myself why I wanted to quit.

To begin with, I'd only worked in a hospital and I began to realize that I didn't like working there anymore. In addition, my discouragement about nursing had to do with its being primarily a woman's profession. This means that nurses tend to be underpaid for their work (in a 1997 article, *The New York Times* reported that full-time working women's earnings are just under 75 percent of men's), and that caring for people does not have high status in our society. Compare caring, what nurses mainly do, with curing, what doctors mainly do, and you'll see which is the highest paid and carries the most prestige. Aha, I said to myself, you want to quit nursing because of what others think about it.

But, when I delved further inside myself, I knew that nursing, and the work nurses did, was incredibly unique, valuable, and most of all needed. This completely changed my mind as it dawned on me that I wanted to quit a hard job because others didn't necessarily see its value even though I knew it was valuable and, in fact, even essential to human life. I can tell you now, nothing gets my attention like seeing there is something I can do that truly makes a difference—I don't care what anyone thinks.

I've struggled with my choice to be a nurse and eventually made the decision to remain one. Doing this has strengthened my commitment to the profession and, I think, qualified me to help you understand what nursing is and what it is not. Promoting nursing is something of a mission for me, partly because I believe in nursing's valuable service and partly because I don't want nursing care, as traditional women's work, or as just being about caring, to be thought of as second best and brushed aside. Nurses are remarkable people and the work they do is incredibly complex, beneficial, and full of healing power. As public recognition of these qualities increases, equitable salaries and prestige will follow.

Nurses Are Not Doctor Wannabes

I can guarantee you every nurse has heard the following at one time or another: "Why didn't you go on to be a doctor?" "You're so smart; you should be a doctor." "You're just a nurse. Are you going to become a doctor?"

The truth is that while these assumptions may be humiliating, degrading, and hurtful, they also indicate the extent of the misunderstanding that exists about nursing. Can you imagine the reverse? "Doctor, why didn't you go on to be a nurse?" "You're so smart; you should become a nurse." "You're just a doctor. When are you going to become a nurse?" or, best of all, "Doctor, you're so good with patients you should be a nurse!" The absurdity of these makes them quite laughable, but asking a nurse the same questions is not at all out of the ordinary (much less funny) and is a good indicator of how our society sees nurses.

Nurses are often viewed as being beneath doctors, not as different or equal, but as a step lower on the health profession or medical ladder. But nursing is as different from being a doctor as being a physical therapist is from being a pharmacist, or as being a teacher is from being a guidance counselor—both of whom work in the field of education with different roles and licensing requirements; nurses, doctors, pharmacists, and physical therapists also work in the same field doing different kinds of work with unique licenses.

Nurses do not practice medicine, they practice nursing; they do not work in the medical field, they work in health care. Nurses have their own philosophy, theory, and concerns just as doctors and pharmacists have theirs.

Nursing's focus is on the care and health of their patients while the doctor's is on diagnosis and cure. This is a big difference. If you are interested in diseases, their causes, and how to get rid of or cure them, then medicine might be for you. If you are more interested in working and caring for people to help them regain or maintain their health, then nursing might be for you.

The two professions do, however, overlap—oftentimes doctors care and nurses cure. You see nurses diagnosing an ear infection and writing a prescription for an antibiotic to cure that infection just as you see a doctor provide comfort and care by quietly holding the hand of a dying patient.

Please keep this in mind. You must analyze what each health profession does and then ask yourself: Is this what I want to do? Do not pick nursing as a career that's second best to being a doctor. Choose nursing because it lets you do what you want to do. Not because of what others think or because of what you don't know—yet.

What Students Making Career Choices Think

If you read research studies about what students think of nursing as a career, you'll see that few even think about it, much less go into it. In a study of high school sophomores, less than 28 percent of those planning to attend college considered nursing as a career option, and of those, only 7 percent actually pursued it. One reason for these low numbers is that nursing is often not presented to students as a choice, and if it is, it is misrepresented.

The six top reasons students give for not considering nursing as a career are: (1) nursing school is too difficult and costly; (2) nursing school is too difficult and not worth it later in terms of salary and status; (3) nurses don't receive enough respect, power, or leadership opportunities; (4) nurses work too hard and do manual labor; (5) nurses are not appreciated; and (6) students disliked the idea of being around people who were dying.

On the other hand, the top seven reasons students gave for considering nursing were: (1) nurses care for and help other people; (2) nurses work with people who have illnesses; (3) there are many professional opportunities; (4) nurses have job security; (5) nursing is nurturing; (6) students surveyed liked science; and (7) the profession of nursing has many personal benefits. In short, students like the idea of caring for others, using their intelligence, and learning about science, but they want more power, less hard work, and a good salary for their efforts.

We'll talk about all of these issues in this book, but for starters, nurses make a very good salary—unless you compare them with other health professionals such as doctors, some physical therapists, pharmacists, and others in health care, many of whom make more than nurses. The average starting salary for a new RN in a hospital is $30,000 while the average income for all RNs is $42,071. Compare this with the salary of a new doctor, or resident, who makes an average of $30,000 and then goes on to average a net income of $195,500.

Nurses have a great deal of responsibility—they literally hold the lives and well-being of others in their hands—so, while the pay is excellent in terms of providing a good living, it is not as good in terms of comparable worth. It all depends on your perspective. Start thinking about salary as one of your reasons for wanting to be or not wanting to be a nurse (add it to your pros and cons list) and, remember, that is the question, at least in this book.

What Do You Think of When You Think of a Nurse

So what do you think? What is your image of a nurse? If you are thinking of nursing as a career, it is critical that you start clarifying your concept of nursing. You don't want to miss the opportunity of a lifetime by rejecting nursing on the basis of false impressions. Likewise, you don't want to waste your time going into nursing for reasons that don't match reality.

Take a moment. When you think of a nurse what do you see? I'll bet it doesn't take you long to come up with a picture. Maybe someone in your family is a nurse. You've certainly seen nurses in the movies or on TV. Shows like *Chicago Hope* and *ER* portray nurses, or at least the networks' idea of nurses, as do the real-life enactment shows like *Rescue 911*. Maybe you've been in a hospital, or had a family member or friend in one. Perhaps a grandparent has had a home health nurse, or has recently been in a nursing home.

Close your eyes and picture "a nurse." What does your nurse look like? Is your nurse a she or a he? Does your nurse have on a white hat and white uniform? Surgical scrubs? Is your nurse holding a gigantic dripping hypodermic syringe or a bedpan? Is your nurse dressed in street clothes with a stethoscope?

Next picture what your nurse is doing. Is she or he feeding a baby or delivering one? Obeying a doctor's orders or giving orders? Standing quietly by while a doctor or priest discusses dying with a patient and family, or doing the talking while the doctors watch? Is this nurse in a hospital or in a clinic? In someone's home or flying in a helicopter? Changing sheets or prescribing medications?

I hope you're thinking, because before we can really talk about what it takes to become a nurse you need to know something about what a nurse is. You may already have a clear idea, and if so, you're one of the lucky few.

Are You Considering Nursing for the Right Reasons?

Rebecca Sternberg, a nursing student in her last semester of school, told me, "I didn't really know what I was getting into when I started nursing school. I thought I'd just learn how to help people. It's turned out to be so different from that. Sure, I've learned about helping people, but I've learned so much more. And it's been a lot of hard work."

Rebecca wanted to help people and she knew that's what nurses did and she was right, but only partly so. She had no idea of the extent of information on diseases, drugs, math, nursing theory, communication, and assessment she would have to learn. She almost dropped out, but with the help of her professors, and most of all, her own determination, she worked hard, graduated, and now works as an RN in geriatrics.

Karin Anderson, a high school student living in a rural area north of Spokane, Washington, wanted to be a nurse ever since she had seen Pat Port, RN, save the life of her mother and her unborn brother. Realizing her pregnant mother was about to deliver four weeks early, Karin called the local paramedics. When they arrived on the scene, they immediately saw the seriousness of the situation and called for help. Pat, an experienced and skilled neonatal nurse, who works on the mother-baby team of a helicopter ambulance service, flew out with the pilot and a respiratory therapist to Karin's home in the country. Pat stabilized her patient and successfully transported the mother into the hospital for a safe delivery.

Karin was so impressed by Pat—by her confidence, her skill, and her gentle reassuring manner—that she decided then and there that this was something she wanted to do. Karin has a long way to go to reach the level of nursing that Pat practiced, but it is not out of her reach. Many students, like Karin, decide on nursing after an encounter with a real nurse in a real-life situation. They see the authority and power these nurses have, and they see nursing as something to aspire to.

Joe Adams has been a nurse for twenty years. He went into nursing after being a medic in the Vietnam War. He told me that becoming a nurse was a decision he made because of his Vietnam experiences. He wanted a career in the medical field, but not as a doctor, because he wanted to spend more time with his patients: talking, comforting, and teaching them, as well as helping them make connections when needed through community resources. He decided to work in emergency care as a nurse.

I asked him what he would tell someone who was thinking about going into nursing today. He said, "I'd tell them to think very carefully about it first."

I asked him why, and he explained, "Nursing isn't like it used to be. You can't just go to school and get a job in a hospital right away. It's not as easy as it used to be. You have to be motivated and know what you want to do and set goals."

Then I asked him, "How can a student possibly know what she or he wants to do?" He advised, "Tell her or him to volunteer, or spend a day in an area she or he is interested in—say, the emergency department or a health clinic."

I've heard this advice over and over from other nurses. They emphatically suggest that anyone considering nursing observe what nurses do and talk to them. Ask nurses questions like "How do you organize and prioritize your work each day?" "How do you know when a patient needs help?'' The thinking process behind the answers to these questions is a big part of nursing and by asking them you'll start to find out what goes on in a nurse's head, and thus what the work is really about.

Spend time going to the places you are interested in. The nurses who work there will very likely welcome you. Remember: Call ahead and explain that you want to see what they do in their job because you are interested in becoming a nurse. Tell them that you want more firsthand experience so that you can be sure before you commit to the nursing profession.

Another option is to volunteer. Many hospitals, clinics, and nursing homes have volunteer positions. Volunteering gives you an excellent firsthand look at what nurses do, as well as giving you an opportunity to meet and talk with them.

Are You Avoiding Nursing for the Wrong Reasons?

A friend of mine has a daughter who is graduating as valedictorian from high school this year. She told me that her daughter had talked about going into nursing out of a desire to work in health care and because she was interested in science and liked working with people. Even though these were perfectly good reasons for going into nursing, she decided against it because it lacked prestige. Instead she decided to become a medical technician and work in a hospital laboratory.

This is an example of deciding not to go into nursing for the wrong reasons. Though nursing may be perceived as lacking prestige, studies show that people who have been hospitalized think nurses are the most important people there. To the people who have been cared for by a nurse, the nurse is a problem solver, a comfort giver, a skilled troubleshooter, and a real lifesaver. Don't forget that nursing's image is changing. Nurses and their professional associations are campaigning hard to show people what nurses really do. The American Nurses Association even has full-time media personnel especially for this purpose.

Health care is changing as well and new nursing opportunities such as nurse practitioner, midwife, and researcher are growing roles. The prestige and authority of nurses is changing and growing just as fast. This is a golden time for nursing, and although we are having bumpy times along with the rest of health care, we are at a point of great positive change and great positive energy. This will go a long way toward improving the image of nursing that makes it seem less of an attractive career than it really is.

Do You Know What You Want to Be
When You Grow Up?

It's not uncommon to never want to grow up, but that doesn't mean you don't have to decide what you are going to do for a living. It does mean that you may change careers as you go along, which is exactly what more and more people are doing these days; many people come to nursing from other careers (see Chapter 3).

If, however, you are younger, you may be deciding for the first time what you want to do. In some ways it's like going fly-fishing—casting your line here and there, looking for a good spot, hoping one of those deep pools that you know must be full of fish and opportunity lies just around the next corner.

On the other hand, you may be able to say, "I've always known I wanted to be a nurse." If this is the case, you can use this book's advice to make sure you do so for the right reasons and to make critical decisions about your education.

If you don't know for sure, then this book will go a long way toward helping you make a decision. As a nurse, I am qualified to tell you that asking the question "What do I want to be when I grow up?" is healthy. Asking it throughout your life puts you on a lifelong learning curve that will keep your mind and soul in excellent shape. And, as you know, a healthy mind promotes a healthier body.

Your assignment, then, is to think about your concepts of nursing, the images of nurses you see portrayed on TV and in books. Compare them with reality. Then decide whether you want to be a nurse. Start out with the following exercise. Make a list, or draw a picture, of your typical nurse. Consider the gender, age, personality, and type of work your nurse is doing. Don't forget to include what you think and feel about all this. For example, your nurse might be carefully assisting an elderly person with his or her insulin injections. Do you think of this in a positive way?

Angels of Mercy and Other Mythical Creatures

Nursing is not short of one thing, and that is stereotypes. Examples include Florence Nightingale as an angel of mercy; the sexy war nurse, just as Hemingway may have pictured her, on the cover of pulp paperbacks; or as a vindictive sneering Nurse Ratched harassing Jack Nicholson in *One Flew Over the Cuckoo's Nest*.

One classic stereotype was conjured up in 1843 by Charles Dickens in

Martin Chuzzlewit. In it we are introduced to Sarah Gamp: midwife, home nurse, and "layer-out of the dead." She was mainly a comic figure, but also uneducated, unprincipled, and a drunk. The image of Sarah Gamp the nurse remains alive today and is considered by nursing historians a frighteningly accurate portrayal of the mid-nineteenth-century nurse. Others give the Sarah Gamps of the nineteenth century more credit by arguing that these nurses practiced their profession independently and were far more clinically proficient than physicians of the day. Whether the portrayal of Sarah Gamp is historically accurate or not, it certainly underscores how fictional characters can affect our thinking.

Stories about women have frequently centered on male characters, romances, and marriages, while neglecting personal achievements and rewards. Nurses are no exception and indeed have provided ample fodder for the pulp fiction mill. Nurses are portrayed in gender and sexual conflicts, as mothers, sisters, sexual temptresses, or, in the reverse, as lonely, cold spinsters who work solely to fill the void of an unhappy life. Rarely are they portrayed as proficient, educated, caring professionals.

The depiction of nurses in fiction shows how our culture regards them. Many stories portray nurses first as vulnerable women and second as skilled workers. One of my personal favorites is a paperback titled *Big City Nurse* with the reading line "The thrilling story of a young nurse's difficult decision—career or love, security or the inner satisfaction of serving humanity." This, of course, implies that nurses cannot do both —unlike the male doctors they fall in love with, who seem quite capable of being husbands, lovers, and saviors of humanity, all at the same time.

Another book I get a laugh out of (and let me add that it has taken me a long time to appreciate the cultural significance of these books with humor, because they used to completely offend me) is called *The New Nurse*. The question the author asks us on the cover is "Could her dedication as a nurse conquer the passion of her woman's heart?" That kind of thinking leads down the path of seeing nurses as mere abstractions, virtuous and pure, who must decide between work and a life of immorality; like Eve and the story of the Fall, they must not give in to desire and thereby forsake humanity. Don't forget, it is usually a doctor who is seen as the target of the young nurse's passions; they, however, are not seen as equally culpable or immoral.

A few more examples that may or may not come from tacky paperbacks include the woman in white who stands when the doctor enters the room and submissively takes orders, or who silently floats through long hospital corridors placing cool cloths on feverish brows. These are all myths, but it just so happens one part is true: nurses do give comfort and a great deal of it.

Not all the images we see are misleading. A picture of a Vietnam nurse working long hours to save lives; the image of a nurse providing care and comfort in the home of a dying patient and family; a nurse caring for a premature baby not much bigger than a fist. These are heroic images, very different from the ones in fiction. They show nurses doing their work for the sake of that work, not for finding a husband, being a martyr, or playing a bossy matron.

Before I became a nurse, or even thought of becoming one, I didn't know about the heroic images, only the negative stereotypes. Nursing didn't appeal to me at all, nor did it seem exciting or challenging. I had no idea what it took to be a nurse. All I knew was that nurses wore white, were mostly women, followed someone else's orders, usually a man's, and worked with sick people in hospitals. I did not like hospitals, I did not like being around sick people, and I did not want to take orders, especially from a man.

When I was twenty-three I was working as a counselor with a woman named Dale at a family planning clinic in Massachusetts. Dale was quitting her job as the manager of volunteers to go to nursing school and I was shocked. Why would Dale, so smart, so down-to-earth and independent, want to be a nurse? Well, I never asked her that question, but I did see her again about a year later. She said she loved nursing school and was excited about being there. She looked the same, dressed the same, talked the same. "Hmmm," I thought to myself, "maybe there is something to nursing that I don't know about."

Later that year I began working as a clinic assistant in a neighborhood health center run by nurse practitioners. These nurses were amazing, they acted so differently from my previous concepts. They did complete health exams, diagnosed problems, and prescribed treatments. They acted with confidence and kindness in talking to the clients and answering all their questions about their illnesses and about taking care of their bodies. I never asked them any questions about being a nurse, mainly because I was shy and easily intimidated, and because I thought they knew so much and I so little. But I found it all very interesting, and I began to form a new, more realistic image of nursing.

It was quite a few years later before I actually went to nursing school, but the seeds were planted back in the health center. So, you see, stereotypes can be changed through observation of real nurses. One study of nursing students found that the biggest influence on their decision to go into nursing was having a family member who was a nurse. So start looking. Whom do you know, whom can you ask, or, in this case, what can you read? I'm a real nurse and I can tell you what real nurses do.

Real Nurses Are Real People

Information, such as where nurses work, what they do, who they are, and how much money they make, can enhance your understanding of the nursing profession and, in turn, help you make a career decision. Thus, in this section I have included statistics on nursing demographics from the American Nursing Association, the National Bureau of Labor, the U.S. Department of Health and Human Services, and the American Association of Colleges of Nursing.

Nursing is the largest health profession in the United States. There are over 2.5 million nurses and, of these, 82.7 percent are employed and working as nurses. More nurses than ever are working full-time: 71.4 percent work full-time and 28.6 percent work part-time.

Non-Caucasian RNs make up only 10 percent of all nurses: 4.2 percent are African-American (non-Hispanic), 3.4 percent are Asian/Pacific Islander, 1.6 percent are Hispanic, and 0.5 percent are Native American or Alaskan Native. As recruitment efforts increase there will be more diversity among nurses.

Over 94 percent of nurses are women. In 1996, 5 percent of nurses were men but this number is growing. In 1996, nursing schools reported that up to 12–13 percent of their students are men.

The average salary for nurses in all settings is $42,071, an 11 percent increase since 1992. The average salary for a staff nurse in a hospital is $40,097, a 9.5 percent increase since 1992. Nurses with advanced practice, or graduate, degrees can earn $80,000–$90,000 or more a year. Approximately 6–7 percent of all registered nurses work as advanced practice nurses. These include nurse practitioners, nurse midwives, clinical nurse specialists, and nurse anesthetists.

The average age of a nurse is forty-four. Sixty percent of nurses are between the ages of 30 and 49. The average age of a new nurse is 33. Many enter nursing as a second career; close to 30 percent of RNs previously worked in other health care positions. Eight percent of these RNs had other college degrees before entering nursing.

The majority of nurses work in hospitals. About two-thirds, or 60 percent, of all nurses work in hospitals today, but by the year 2000 that is expected to drop to one-half as more health care services are being offered in outpatient clinics, in homes, in community centers, and in nursing homes. In the past, most newly graduated RNs' first job was in a hospital. Now, as jobs in hospitals decrease, there are more new graduates going to work in community settings like nursing homes.

Health Care Is Changing

Health care costs have grown outrageously and, in an attempt to bring them down, providing care for less money has become an important issue. As a result, new systems of delivering health care have evolved. You've probably heard of managed care or of HMOs (health maintenance organizations). These systems are designed to provide health care to people for less money by carefully managing their patients. Keeping people healthy is one goal, as is minimizing hospital stays when they are sick.

Hospitals are expensive places to provide health care because they require large numbers of staff and equipment. That's one reason why so many surgeries and procedures that used to require several days in the hospital are being done in one day through outpatient clinics. Examples include cataract surgery for the eyes and orthopedic procedures such as knee surgery. Having your gallbladder removed used to mean a week or more in the hospital. Now, because of new technology, it can be safely done in one day for a lot less money.

Nursing research is contributing to finding ways to provide quality health care for less cost. This research supplies evidence for making important health care decisions which in turn results in better care for patients. In many cases, these practices are replacing old ways of doing things—ways that were expensive and not necessarily better for the patients.

One important advance, disease prevention, is something nurses have been working on for over a hundred years. If we can help people improve their health, there will be fewer illnesses requiring expensive hospitalization. Helping people quit smoking or eat a nutritious diet, for instance, can have immense effects on health in terms of lung and heart disease, prenatal health, and many other conditions. Nurses want to save money, but nursing's number one concern is that people lead healthy lives and receive the best health care (health care that meets their needs, and not the needs of someone else's pocketbook).

In a dramatic shift from the past, health care is moving away from treating illnesses after they occur and, instead, turning toward health and wellness. Nursing has always focused on health promotion and disease prevention. As far back as 1889, Florence Nightingale herself predicted this turn toward wellness. She said that by the year 2000 hospitals would be obsolete because nurses would be working to keep people well. Although it is unlikely that this prediction will fully come to pass, she was right that nurses would be working hard to keep people healthy.

Again, it is just common sense. Why not have a nurse managing people with diseases, or who are at risk for disease, by teaching, counseling, assessment, and coordination of their care? It costs much less money for a nurse to help a patient with heart failure, diabetes, or asthma to stay healthy than to wait for that patient to get sick enough to go to the emergency room and wind up in the hospital.

There will continue to be a need for hospitals for the critically ill—nurses will continue to work in emergency, intensive care, surgery, oncology, and psychiatric units just as they do now. But the main focus of health care will be on prevention and management of diseases in the home, the community, and internationally, and this is precisely what the philosophy of the nursing profession is all about.

The following are some of the population trends affecting health care today. Nurses are responding to these trends by expanding their roles and by revising nursing school curriculums to teach students what they will need to know to be effective nurses in the twenty-first century.

People Are Living Longer

The number of older people, called an "aging population," is increasing. If you're in high school or college, your parents are probably baby boomers and they will be making up this segment of the population. As more advances are made in technology and treatment of diseases, people are living longer. As a result, we will see more chronic illnesses, like heart disease and diabetes. People will want to live in their own homes as long as possible and remain active (this is especially going to be true of the baby boomers who like to ski, travel, kayak, etc.). Nurses have always been experts on managing chronic illnesses—helping people to stay fit and healthy while living in their own homes—so this trend has a positive effect on nursing jobs.

Everything Costs Too Much and
We Don't Like It Anyway

Everyone has heard about the health care crises; about rising costs and the desperate need to reduce them, and about a general dissatisfaction with health-care services. Although health care reform headed up by Hillary Rodham Clinton was killed in the early 1990s, reducing cost remains a hot social and legislative issue. Reducing cost is important to nurses because we want to provide quality health care for as many people as possible. In fact, study after study shows that the number one concern of RNs is quality of care. As insurers and providers alike work to improve customer satisfaction, nurses will be called upon to work in quality management, outcomes research, and public relations.

People Want Help Being Healthy

Overall, we are seeing a change in health care from just treating disease and illness after they happen to trying to prevent them. The focus is more on keeping people well, and yes, while this is driven by a need to reduce money spent on health care, it is an important shift in the way we run our health care system. As I just discussed, nurses have worked in health promotion and disease prevention for over one hundred years. Many nurses today work in preventive programs such as nutrition, exercise, and weight management.

People Are Demanding More Information

Gone are the days when people simply did what the doctor ordered. We all want to know about the medications we take and about any tests we need. Nurses have always been the ones to inform people and help them make decisions. This is a trend that is good for everyone as well as for nursing. People need to be informed so they can take responsibility for their health.

So Many People—So Little Health Care

This is a big problem. Many people, especially women and children, have no health insurance. Often this is because they don't have any money. Nurses have taken political action to change laws and make policies to help people get health care. Nurses have increased the number of children in our country that are immunized against childhood diseases, advocated for children and others living in poverty, and supported safety issues such as gun control. This kind of work is part of nursing's history: nurses started the first public health centers and homes for the poor, called settlement houses.

Access to health care is a huge issue, and you could go into nursing just to work on that problem alone! After all, what's the use of having an excellent health care sysem if only some of the people get to use it? This trend has a negative impact not only on nursing jobs but on everyone else. When families without insurance get sick they may not be able to work. If they have to go on public assistance we pay more as taxpayers than if their employers, or government, paid their insurance benefits. Not only that, but families and individuals under stress are much more prone to illness and injury—further driving up costs.

But enough politics for now—the purpose of this book is to help you understand what a nurse is, what it takes to be a nurse, if you want to become one, and if so, how to go about it. So let's get going. No blood, no guts, but lots of glory.

▪ 2 ▪

Tell Someone Who Cares

"Nurses have the courage to care." This was the 1997 National Nurses' Day motto, and something people say over and over about nurses. My friend's fifteen-year-old daughter Alisha told me, "Someone who is going to be a nurse has to be a caring person." She's right, but what does it mean to care?

Compassion, knowledge, honesty, and confidence are components of caring, according to nursing theory, which states that caring is "the essence" of nursing practice. You probably have your own ideas. You care about a friend, you care about how you look and feel, you care for a pet, you care about your family. You could say caring means that you have good feelings for someone or something, that you want them to do well, and that you may even love them.

Here's what a group of senior nursing students had to say about caring:

"Caring means giving close attention."

"Giving of yourself."

"To be helpful and nurturing."

"Caring is being concerned."

"Caring is the same as meeting needs."

Caring is thinking about what you would want for yourself or for your family and then, as many nurses do, using that to guide you in your work, even when the pressure is on: the workload is heavy, you're tired, there is too much to do in too little time, but as a nurse you will be thinking, "What would I want for this patient if he or she were my mother, my child, or me?"

For example, when Sharon Reynolds was a new nurse working in a small hospital she took care of a young first-time mother and her husband. It was time for the woman to deliver, but the baby had died before birth. Still, the woman had to go through labor to deliver the baby. Sharon worked overtime into the next shifts caring for this family and helping them physically and emotionally through a very painful experience. She said, "I just kept thinking about what I would want and need if I was the one going through that. When I got so tired and felt overwhelmed myself with the tragedy, this kept me going."

Caring is a nursing value. Values guide your work and your life; they provide a foundation for your actions. Other nursing values include: compassion, advocacy, respect for the rights and beliefs of others, justice, knowledge, and honesty. Caring is manifest in all sorts of ways, not just between a nurse and patient or family. Carol Bonnono, RN, is an emergency department (ED) nurse in Oregon who cared enough about accident victims of drunk drivers that she went to her state governor about it. Up to the time Carol took action, ED nurses, because of patient privacy rights, were not permitted to report patients with alcohol levels above 0.15 percent to the police. In an article she wrote in the *American Journal of Nursing* (September 1997) she said:

> As an ED nurse, I was outraged when I learned this. I strongly believe ED personnel should not only be allowed but required to inform law officers of patients whose blood alcohol level exceeds legal limits. I was treating the same people week after week for injuries sustained in motor vehicle accidents they caused by driving while intoxicated, and I could do nothing but help stitch them up and send them back out on the road.

Oregon now has a law that changed reporting requirements and, in the first year, they saw a 1 percent reduction in alcohol-related fatalities. On a national level, Oregon congresswoman Elizabeth Furse introduced a bill, House Resolution 1982, which she calls the "Carol Bonnono Bill." Carol, who considers herself a patient advocate like all other nurses, turned her frustration and anger into action motivated by her caring.

Who Cares Who Cures?

Do doctors only cure illness and nurses only care for the people who are ill? The main differences between doctors and nurses are the principles and goals guiding their work. A nurse's primary mission is to care for people before, during, or after episodes of illness. A doctor's is to diagnose and cure illnesses. These basic premises form the foundation of each profession's practice, but they do not limit it. For instance, nurses often diagnose and cure illnesses, while doctors care for and comfort their

patients. This overlap of roles leads to confusion about the distinct in-
dividuality of the two professions.

Nurses do many things to help people get over an illness. Nurse practitioners can diagnose health problems and prescribe medications to treat
those problems. For instance, Cherrie Takenaka, a nationally certified
family nurse practitioner with a master's degree in nursing, has prescription authority in the state of Washington. (This authorization to prescribe
drugs varies from state to state.) She works in an office with a family
doctor, has her own patients, diagnoses their problems, and prescribes
treatments. When she needs help she talks with the doctor, consults with
a specialist or refers the patient to one.

Curing is easier to describe than caring (which is one very good reason
why nursing is hard to define). Think of a time when you felt cared for
or when you cared for someone else. Would it be hard to describe that
experience? A student in one of my classes, Nancy Wilimek, described
caring by telling a story about a patient she was assigned to. She was
going in to assess him after he had a CAT scan to look for lung cancer.
Although he appeared to be resting quietly in bed, she only had to take
one look at him to know he was scared out of his wits. "I looked into
his eyes and saw fear. Fear as plain as day. He was absolutely petrified.
So I sat down next to him, took his hand, and asked him how he was.
He began to cry. I continued to hold his hand, and he cried for a while.
He told me that I was the first person that day to pay any attention to
him."

The man had been in the hospital all day getting tests, interacting with
doctors, technicians, hospital personnel, and other nurses, and at the end
of the day he felt that Nancy was the first to pay attention to him, as a
person, not just as a case. Nancy understood that he was vulnerable and
in a scary situation. By letting him express his fear, she cared for him in
a way that no one else did, and with what we know today about mind-
body interactions, caring can be part of the cure.

Another nursing student, Karen Huffman, described caring like this:

> When my grandfather was in the hospital the nurses were the
> ones that were there all the time. They were interested in us and
> how we felt. When he went home they made sure we had all the
> information we needed. The doctors, on the other hand, came in
> and out of the room. Checked Grandpa briefly and left. The nurses
> were the most important to us.

Alisha experienced caring after an injury in ballet class:

When I went to the emergency room with a twisted ankle the nurse was very nice. He talked to me and told me everything he was doing. He taught me how to take care of my ankle. He was good, they all are. And I've mainly had all men nurses when I've gone in.

Another way to think about caring is to think about comfort. Research has shown that making patients comfortable is essential to good nursing care. Researcher Katherine Kolcaba, RN, PhD, put it this way:

We have long recognized that comfortable patients heal faster, cope better, become rehabilitated more thoroughly, or die more peacefully than do the uncomfortable. Patient comfort is the essence of nursing and contributes to patients' quality of life.

Who's Who in the Health Care Zoo?

Health care is a term that covers everything from nursing to medicine to homeopathy. To better understand nursing you have to understand the place of different professions within the health care system. Health care professionals do all sorts of things to help people improve their health, whether they are sick or not. Think of going for a sports physical. You're not sick, but you need to be checked to make sure it is safe for you to play sports.

On the other hand, you may be very sick with a bacterial infection in your throat. In this case you get health care that will, hopefully, cure your sickness. Another example is going to a clinic to check for sexually transmitted diseases. This is a routine visit and you may not be sick at all. You will receive information and have your questions answered by experts in that field. If you have a disease, you will receive treatment. These types of exams, education, and treatment can be provided by nurses or doctors.

Nurses can do all the things listed above: giving sports physicals, educating patients, treating infections, and answering questions. Doctors do, too. The key point is that nursing and medicine are different professions with different focuses. For instance, doctors diagnose and treat diseases; nurses promote health, educate and care for families. Think of a physical therapist, a dentist, an acupuncturist, a registered dietitian, and a social worker. These people are all in health care professions. But their jobs are all different.

More confusing are the differences between RNs, LPNs, and PAs. LPNs, or licensed practical nurses, have one year of training, most often work in hospitals and nursing homes, and perform less complicated work than RNs. Physician's assistants are commonly confused with nurse practitioners. Nurse practitioners, RNs who have obtained a graduate degree in nursing, usually practice under their state's nursing board. Physician's assistants, or PAs, usually, but not always, have previous health care experience, say as a medic in the military, and then attend a program that is one to two years in length. PAs work under the physician's license. (For more on nurse practitioners, see Chapter 7.)

Nurses receive an extraordinary education that gives them the unique and broad view needed to treat the whole person (this is also referred to as holistic healing). While studying nursing in college, you will take classes in the humanities, such as education, multicultural studies, and fine arts, in addition to sciences like pathophysiology and pharmacology. Nurses also need political knowledge to work on making changes that will improve health care services; courses such as psychology and history to help them work with diverse populations; and sociology to help solve family and other social problems such as domestic violence and meeting the unique needs of elders or teenagers.

Again, this is why it is hard to describe nursing—there is so much to it—and at the same time why nursing has so many fascinating opportunities. At this point you should be starting to see that nursing is not what you thought, or perhaps that it includes more than you thought. Nursing is not just a chance to get a quick job in a hospital helping people feel better. Nursing is about a commitment to knowledge and, as a professional, to learning whatever you need to care for and cure people.

A Woman's Work Is Never Done: But Who Cares!

Before Florence Nightingale appeared on the scene in the mid-nineteenth century, women were responsible for taking care of sick family members in the home. This was because hospitals used to be terribly unsanitary places where patients, three to four to a bed, went to die rather than to be healed. Knowledge about many diseases, especially infectious diseases, was lacking.

Florence Nightingale, the most famous nurse in history, used her talent and knowledge acquired in the Crimean War to reform hospitals. Some of her most important work had to do with the design and management of hospitals based on her theory that, in a proper environment, nature could heal. Her theory holds true today. Cleanliness, fresh air, and good nutrition are things that nurses use today to promote health and prevent illness.

Florence Nightingale ended up portrayed as an angel of mercy, and she has largely been remembered for this image rather than for her work as a nurse. Nightingale was born into a rich, educated English family, received an excellent education, and traveled extensively. Her biggest problem was that she wanted to do meaningful work. This was a problem because women of her day, especially upper-class women, did not work outside the home. If a woman did, it was usually out of necessity—in other words, poverty. As a wealthy, educated woman, Florence was expected to get married. Period.

She had to choose between doing what her family wanted and becoming a nurse. Today, this would not be such a difficult decision. But for her, it meant a choice between giving up what she wanted and being alienated from and, possibly, disowned by her family. Florence left her family to become a nurse and for many years had no contact with her mother or sister. Her writing shows how painful this was for her, but she considered her work important enough to put up with it.

In 1854, Nightingale was asked by the British government to go to the Crimea, where England was at war. She was excited about this opportunity, but probably had no idea what she was getting into. She was shocked and horrified by the conditions she found the soldiers living in, both the injured and the healthy. There was no sanitation, raw sewage water was used in cooking, and drinking water was contaminated by animal carcasses that lay in the streams.

She organized and restructured the camps and, in doing so, saved the lives of thousands. Late at night she wrote letters to the government that resulted in radical changes, and she is credited with being the most effective person in British history in improving the status and treatment of the British soldier.

Nightingale also kept detailed records of what happened during her time in the Crimea. She recorded the number of men who lived and died, and the number and types of their injuries, and, as such, became the first biostatistician (someone who records statistics on humans). After her outstanding work in the Crimea, she was a worldwide heroine. Everyone knew her name, just as they do today.

Eventually she talked to her family again, but she never married. In fact, nurses, like teachers, by law could not marry because having children and making a living by taking care of people were not viewed as compatible. Furthermore, there were no male nurses—you had to be a woman to be a nurse. So nursing was literally and legally women's work and that fact has had a profound impact on the profession, in terms of both salary and image.

Joe, who started out as a medic in Vietnam, told me how he thought it affected his moneymaking ability. "I am very aware of nursing as woman's work and that it is thought of that way. Women always take care of people, especially sick people. They are expected to do it. It is supposed to come naturally. That's why we don't get paid as much for what we do."

Theo Alkin, RN, working in a large emergency department, pointed out similarly how it affects image: "Nurses, because we are women, are expected to do all the things we do. It is supposed to come naturally. People don't think as highly about what we do. We just do it."

What this means to you as a potential nurse is that you'll inherit some problems. It is no news that women make less money than men. Lower pay is generally connected to work that involves caring for others, like nursing and teaching. It's no surprise that others in the health care field make more than nurses. Ask yourself these questions: Why do doctors get paid so much more than nurses? Why do doctors have more prestige than nurses?

An obvious answer would be that, traditionally, nurses are women and doctors are men. Or you could say it is because society values the type of work doctors do, curing, over what nurses do, caring. Take a look at a magazine or newspaper article about health care, and you will see that doctors are the main feature. Likewise, when I see a preview of a show on TV that's going to be about health care, I know that it will be about doctors, and 99 percent of the time I am right. One study showed that literature on health policy and issues rarely mentions nurses despite the fact that nurses make up the largest group of health care providers.

Another answer to these questions is that doctors have more responsibility than nurses. But how do you define responsibility? Does a teacher who spends the entire day, day after day, with a young child developing a lifetime of learning have as much responsibility as a doctor who sees that same child for five minutes about an earache? Does a nurse who manages the medications and care of twenty patients have less responsibility than a doctor who performs the removal of a gallbladder? As a society, we say that the doctor has more responsibility and therefore more value.

Responsibility and value are defined by individuals and by society. I think some of these definitions are changing, though (and if I have anything to do with it they will). Promotion of health, a professional responsibility of nursing, is gaining status, and likewise, RNs are beginning to be recognized for their work. But this recognition has largely been our own doing. Instead of meekly waiting for someone to come along and notice us, we're out on the street corners shouting our

own praise and in research laboratories crunching numbers to statisti-
cally show the value of our work.

In nursing, a high level of technical and clinical skills combine with
caring skills to provide comfort and save lives. Pat, a neonatal flight
nurse, demonstrated this late one night as she transported a critical new-
born via helicopter from a small hospital to a larger medical center.

One night we went to transport a ventilator-dependent baby with
a massive pulmonary hemorrhage. The baby was in critical condition, so we also brought her mother on board. I wanted the mother
to see that I was doing all I could for her baby—not everyone will
do that, but that is important to me. Coming back to the hospital
the weather was really crappy. The rain and wind were so strong
we were blown around like a rag doll. The pilot was unable to even
make out the horizon. All the lights on board the helicopter had to
be turned off so the pilot could navigate by street and car lights
below. The only light we had to work with was from the monitor,
and even that had to be screened from the pilot.

Suddenly, I noticed on the monitor that the baby's oxygen was
dropping quickly. I got out my flashlight and began searching for
clues. Immediately I could see that the baby was bleeding from her
mouth so badly that it caused the security tape on the breathing
tube to come loose. The tube had slipped out of the baby's mouth.
She quickly became symptomatic, with her blood pressure dropping
and heart rate going way up. It's in these kinds of situations where
we flight nurses look at a monitor, see something happen, and ask
ourselves, "What does this mean?" On top of that, we have to work
it through very quickly, determine what to do, and then do it fast.

Here we were, up in the air, we couldn't turn on the lights, and
the only light I had was this little flashlight that I held in my mouth
while I went to work. The baby was lying on her side in the Isolette,
bleeding profusely from the mouth. On top of that we had the
mother on board, so we really had no room to move around. The
baby's mother realized something had gone wrong, but she really
didn't know what was happening. She sat in her jump seat with
terror in her eyes and tears running down her face.

The baby needed to be reintubated (her breathing tube had to be
put back in), but I couldn't see how it could be done in this predicament. Intubation is complicated under the best conditions, especially with infants. All of these thoughts ran through my head in a
fraction of a second. Still, I was left with no choice. In the darkness,
I reached both arms into the portholes of the Isolette. With one

gloved finger, I blindly lifted up the epiglottis (at the back of the baby's throat). With the other hand, I guided a new tube into the airway. It worked, and immediately the vital signs stabilized.

We got to the hospital and the baby and mother eventually went home. The mother was exceptionally grateful that I had the skills to handle that crisis and that she could be there while I cared for her baby.

We Care Too: Men in Nursing

In my nursing research class, I had a male student, Paul Hill, who had long hair and two earrings, drove a motorcycle, and worked in a hospital emergency department. He was twenty-six years old and had just gotten married. As the semester progressed, I asked him why he had become a nurse.

"My mother wanted me to," he joked. "She's a nurse, but when I was thinking about what to do after high school, nursing seemed a good option. I liked science and I was interested in health. I thought it would be a good job to learn in, and one that I could keep learning in."

One day in class we talked about conflict in the workplace when one of the students described her attempts to persuade hospital administrators that more nurses were needed on her unit to safely take care of patients. The administrators responded, "We don't have the money. Make do with what you have." Feeling extremely frustrated by the interaction and, because the hospital had lately been laying off RNs, the student didn't feel secure in further discussion, much less confrontation.

Paul listened carefully and said, "That's when you need the support of other nurses: to make your point with a unified voice. If people don't like it, don't act rude or anything, but don't back down."

I liked that. This sums up a great deal of what nursing is about today. Nurses have to be able to work together for change in an environment that does not always favor what the nurses think. Nurses think first about quality of care. To work in health care today, one needs skill and the ability to negotiate and come to agreeable compromises. Paul was able to pinpoint the problem.

Nurses do things that both men and women can do. There is nothing about nursing, except our image of it, that makes it necessary to be a woman. Caring, communicating, making decisions, working for health —these are all things both men and women can do.

Only 5 percent of all nurses are men, but that is rapidly changing as the number of men going to nursing school increases. In 1996, 12–13 percent of nursing school graduates were men, an increase from

11 percent in just one year. From 1980 to 1992, while the total number of RNs increased by only 35 percent, the numbers of male RNs increased by 97 percent.

Why is this? Nursing offers options, challenges, and rewards to both men and women. As our society becomes less focused on outmoded gender roles, everyone's options for work increase. Just as you see women taking on careers traditionally held by men, men are taking careers traditionally held by women. Stereotypes are breaking down, slowly, but they are breaking down. The days when it was a requirement to be a woman in order to become a nurse are long gone.

Men do face problems in nursing, though, and the one most frequently mentioned is "role strain" or pressures related to working in a traditionally female profession. Many men choose to work in emergency or psychiatric departments, or as nurse anesthetists, areas some perceive to be less dominated by women. However, Christine Williams, a University of Texas sociologist, studied men in women's professions and found that men don't get harassed as much as women do for stepping across the gender line; they are promoted faster, and it's more likely men will feel welcomed.

Talking to men in nursing, I was curious whether they faced discrimination or assumptions about their masculinity. Did people see them as less of a man for being a nurse? None of the men I talked to had this problem. Paul said that his older brothers teased him at times, but he said they teased him about everything. He had no problems at work, from either patients or other staff.

I worked with Bill Hughes in the cardiac intensive care unit, and he told me that being a man in nursing meant that some people thought you were the doctor. It's automatic to regard a man as the doctor and a woman as the nurse. He would correct them by saying, "I'm not a doctor, I'm a nurse. I'll be taking care of you and managing your care this evening." He was a favorite of everyone, patients and staff. He was funny, smart, and an excellent nurse.

Another nurse, Bill Harrelson, is a flight nurse for the same air ambulance as Pat Port. The flight service covers over 150 nautical miles and is the fourth largest in the United States. Bill, who loves flight nursing, said he became a nurse because he liked people and science, and he wanted a secure job making a decent amount of money. He has a lot of autonomy in his work; when the team goes on a flight he is in charge of the patient's care. There are no doctors on board or on the radio. Bill decides what to do and how to do it. He's worked hard to get to the point he's at in his career now, but he says it's been worth it, and "I've got the best job in the world."

In Chapter 1, I talked about considering a nursing career for the wrong reasons. Another way to look at this is: "Are you not considering nursing for the wrong reasons?" A survey of college males suggested that if men were given more information about nursing, they would consider it as a career. The primary reason men stay away from nursing is a social one; as long as nursing is thought of as mainly a women's profession, participation by men will continue to be small. If you are a man, and the reason you are not thinking much about nursing is that you think it is a career for women, think again. Don't let your view of gender limit you to a certain type of work. Think about what you want to do and then look at what nursing has to offer in terms of challenges and rewards. Many women have broken into fields previously populated only by men. If women can do it, men can, too.

Caring Means Many Things

Nurses tell stories about their work that show how caring affects their patients. Caring means many things: taking time to listen, advocating for those in need, being open-minded, and making pain relief a priority. Liz McDonald, a home health care nurse, spoke about helping a woman with severe postpartum depression. Her story details how caring involves advocating and being open-minded.

She was so depressed she was talking about leaving her family— her husband and her three kids and new baby. It was really a bad situation. She didn't think she was a good parent, or that she was worth anything at all. I got in touch with her husband and made sure he understood the severity of her depression. I also spoke to her doctor and got her in to see a counselor. Later, when she recovered, she said to me many times, "I really appreciate you because you didn't think of me as a crazy person, you just thought of me as a normal person who was having a hard time. I don't know what would have happened without you."

Theo has been a nurse for twenty years. She is soft-spoken, and appears shy when she talks. She works in the emergency department (ED) of a large regional hospital and trauma center. She talks about how relieving pain is an important aspect of caring.

I had a patient who came to the ED with very painful kidney stones. I worked with her and I said to the doctor and nurses, "You know, we have to get her an IVP [a test for kidney stones], but it needs to wait until I get her pain under control." And that is just routine for me, that's how I do things. I think it's a nice thing to be able to have your pain relieved before you go and have X rays. This is just part of my practice—to relieve someone's pain before they have to go and have more miserable pain.

The next day she sent me flowers. It really made me feel good. I thought, wow, that's really nice, that this person would send me this kind of thing. It doesn't happen often at all, that's why I was so surprised.

With the care of the patient always their first priority, some nurses may stretch a hospital rule here and there. Julie Pyle, working with a young man with cancer, was mainly concerned for his comfort and needs as he was about to die.

He was going to die soon and he so badly wanted to see his little puppy again, so we snuck his puppy into his room for him. If you were really rigid and went strictly by the books, those kinds of things wouldn't be done. But, to me, not to listen to something that was so important to him when he was dying was wrong, too. It really didn't make any difference at all in the grand scheme of things if the puppy came into the hospital. But it made a lot of difference to him, so we did it and it made him smile for the first time in a long time. It was well worth it.

Tell someone who cares? Tell a nurse. Nursing has a century of caring behind it. Caring is like the foundation of a house; it holds all that is built upon it, and shapes and secures it. Caring is nursing's ground, its roots. It holds the profession in place, guiding our work as individually we build our careers and, as a group, our profession.

▪ 3 ▪

Making a Career Decision Is Enough to Make Anyone Sick

Personally, I never really knew what I wanted to be when I grew up, but I had many ideas. When I was very little I wanted to be a beauty queen–movie star, then a psychologist who knew everything in the world. Later I wanted to be a part-time veterinarian, part-time plant pathologist, then a horseshoer-blacksmith-artist, and then . . . well, the list goes on.

Nursing came to me by accident. I worked in many different jobs, but the one I enjoyed most was as a crisis counselor and assistant in a family planning clinic in Massachusetts. I liked talking to people and I was interested in science and in health. And, perhaps more important, I was at a point where I really needed to do something that would not only land me a job but give me one with a good long-term outlook—a career.

As I thought about nursing it seemed to hold potential for the perfect combination of counselor, scientist, and health expert. So, even though, after many years on and off in college, I was only one class away from a degree in biology, I switched majors to nursing and stayed in school for two and a half more years. I even returned to school for two more years after graduating to earn my master's degree in nursing. Being a nurse has turned out to be worth it. It has become much more to me than "a job." Nursing is intriguing, exciting, and a challenge that has taught me at least as much about myself as it has about the world around me.

Growing Up or Throwing Up?

Trying to decide on a career, as you must well know at this point, is not easy. The fear of making a wrong decision is as powerful as your worries about the money, time, and energy needed to reach your goals. What you do for work helps shape your self-image and, as such, is enough to make you a little bit queasy. Whether the butterflies in your stomach are from fear or excitement, or both, ask yourself this question: "Do I picture myself working in a service profession?" If the answer is yes, then congratulations, at least you're on the right track. Nurses, doctors, pharmacists, physical therapists, respiratory therapists, and nutritionists are all members of health professions that offer opportunities to work with and serve other people.

To help you clear your mind and get down to reality, follow these next steps; they will help you answer the question: "What do all these health care professionals really do?"

1. Look at each profession.

What do people in these professions do every day? Do you see yourself doing it? I know people who hate hospitals. They say just the smell makes them sick. Don't rule out a health career for this reason, especially nursing. Many nurses work in clinics, universities, and people's homes. Besides, you can get used to the smell. One teenager told me that the one thing that she thought she would hate about nurses was that they wore very ugly, thick shoes. Unsightly shoes—now there's a reason for a career choice! Not to worry, though, many nurses wear light aerobic shoes or cushioned clogs.

2. Make a list of pros and cons.

If you are thinking of being a medical technician, a pro might be that you'd work with laboratory tests, something you are interested in. A con might be that you'd like working with people more than you'd have an opportunity to as a medical technician, or that you would want to be more flexible in the location of your work.

You might be interested in nursing because you have a desire to help people. A pro would be that most nurses work directly with people. A con might be that changes in health care mean that nurses frequently deal with change—change of work locations, change of policies, change of political views affecting nursing practice. If you don't want that, consider another health care career.

3. Experience the profession firsthand.

This is most important—find someone doing the work you are interested in and ask her to let you follow her around for several weeks, a day, or even just for a few hours (the "anything's better than nothing" approach). This is the best way to get an idea of what really goes on in any job, and the best way to find out if you are really interested in that kind of work or not. Ask your school counselor to help you find someone, or ask a friend or parent who can help you. (See Appendix A for further help.)

Following these steps will help you begin to understand what goes on in the different health professions. Remember, they are all very different.

Some think about health care as an opportunity to find a satisfying career, others as just a place to find a job. Some think of it as both. If you are of the "just find a job" variety, I hope you don't go into nursing for this reason alone. Although I have to admit that I do know a nurse or two who have done so. Luckily, they found out it was work they loved, and went on for more education so that nursing could really become a career for them.

However, I would not recommend this route. Don't become a nurse just to get a job. It is far too demanding a profession for that. First, try to find out if it is what you want to do and you'll save yourself a great deal of hard, frustrating work and heartache. See if you may fit one of the following scenarios, or if you are a combination of several.

Ask yourself these questions about making a nursing career decision: Are you . . .

A. Thinking about what to do after high school to get a job quickly and with reasonable pay?

In this case, if you are thinking of nursing, you are probably thinking of going to community college for a two-year RN program (see Chapter 4). This will be fairly inexpensive and quick. You will find a job in a hospital, or perhaps a clinic, or most likely in an extended care facility like a nursing home. Sound good? There are many reasons to take this option, but remember, if you want to make nursing a career and advance in the profession, you'll need a bachelor's degree in nursing.

I teach in a program for RNs returning to earn their bachelor's degree. They tell me, "I wish I had done it all at once. It would have saved me a lot of time." "I need the four-year degree to get to a higher pay scale." "I need the four-year degree to get a promotion." Other nurses who have found a job they like—in a hospital, for example—are entirely happy with a two-year degree. They are expert clinical nurses, they like where they are, and they plan to stay there.

B. A senior in high school wanting to get a job in health care mainly because you are interested in science?

You're probably thinking about all the different possibilities, including working in a medical laboratory, in respiratory therapy, as a cardiovascular technician, as a nurse, as a doctor, and so on. Your considerations in making a career choice, if you are similar to students in research studies, are: length of schooling, cost of schooling, eventual salary, prestige, authority, and interest in the work.

The obvious choice for the highest salary is becoming a doctor. Prestige, authority, and power all depend on your perspective. Doctors gain automatic rights to these because our society views them that way. Nurses, on the other hand, have these things, but many people don't recognize this side of nursing.

For example, Peggy Clemons, a family nurse practitioner and flight nurse, makes a very good salary, has autonomy and power, and abundant interest in her work. There is also Donna Shertzer, vice president of patient care services at a large urban hospital. She makes decisions that affect hundreds of people, is respected, and makes more than the average hospital nursing administrator's salary of $52,213. Although she no longer practices nursing in a clinical situation, she keeps her license current and considers her nursing experience with patients invaluable in her current job. Jeff Leonard is a nurse anesthetist making about $80,000 a year. He works with an independent group of nurses who contract with hospitals for their services.

You can see that there are nurses who do not conform to the stereotypes, and you don't have to, either. If you have a love of science and you want to work with people, nursing may be for you.

C. Currently going to college and not sure what to do for a career?

You want to study something that will help you find a job, that will be interesting, requires brainpower, offers opportunity for advancement, and gives you some respect and power.

First of all, how good are you in the sciences? Because to be a nurse you'll have to enjoy or learn to enjoy them. Nursing requires daily use of science, especially an understanding of the scientific process. How a nurse thinks and acts is often based on this method of problem solving. To learn how to think like a researcher is important because you must always be asking yourself, "Why am I doing it this way?" "Is this the best for the patient?" "Is it best for the patient and cost-effective?"

Second, do you want to work in health care? Obviously, this is a key point in your decision making. As I've mentioned before, talk to people in the different fields and then observe what they do (see Appendix A).

D. In another job and want to do something different or more interesting?

As I said, almost 30 percent of RNs worked in other health careers before coming to nursing. Many nurses have had other jobs outside of health care, myself included. I worked in family planning, in a research laboratory, and on a farm, to name a few. Peggy worked identifying and cataloging plant species in the wilds of Alaska, as a fish packer, and as a mapmaker. Some of the best nurses have had previous careers. These experiences are valuable and add to your qualifications to become a nurse. (See the next section on second-career RNs.)

E. Majoring in premed?

A seasoned nursing adviser at a large state university told me that many of the students she sees are in the premed program. If so, you may well ask why they were seeing her, the nursing adviser.

These premed students tell her:

"I want to be a doctor, but the science courses required are tougher than I thought they would be."

"I thought I wanted to be a doctor at first. But now I see that I don't, because I don't want to go to school for so long."

Heidi Welch was an excellent high school student from a small farming community where the doctor was very family-oriented. She loved science and saw herself becoming a doctor like the one in her town. She ended up struggling with the science and math classes in college. She thought nursing might be an easier alternative and decided to look into changing majors.

Her adviser told her that nursing was not the same as being a doctor, nor was it easier, but maybe she could still do what she loved and work in a small town. The adviser hooked Heidi up with a nurse practitioner who worked in the country. She was the only health care provider for a large farming and logging community. Heidi followed her around for a few days and found out that this was exactly what she wanted to do. She went back to school, worked with a tutor in the science classes, and changed her major from premed to nursing. This time she did so for the right reason.

Another premed student, James Hall, worked with a physician in a small hospital between his first and second years of college. As he and the doctor went on morning rounds, James began to notice what the nurses did and soon realized that their work was more like what he wanted to do. Why? He said, "I saw that the nurses had far more contact with the patients and their families than the doctor did. The nurses spent more time educating and working on preventive care and that was what I wanted to do." He changed his major from premed to nursing for the right reasons.

James's choice is an example of an excellent reason for changing your major. He observed that nurses were different from doctors and, by comparing the two roles, discovered that he preferred the latter.

In Chapter 1, I talked about stereotypes of nurses and how much of what nurses do is unseen by the casual observer: the thinking process, decision making, evaluating, coordinating, and perhaps most important, the way RNs advocate for the good of the patient and family. Many of the stories in this book show how nurses act as advocates, but perhaps

Liz's story of working in oncology shows best the importance of this unique nursing role, as she advocated for her patient dying from leukemia.

> He was in bad shape—everyone knew he was dying. His platelet count was really low, but he wanted desperately to go home, so I called his hematologist, I think it was a Sunday, and pleaded for him, saying that this guy just wants to go home. But the doctor said, "With his platelet count so low, you know what could happen to him." I said, "Yes, I know, and the patient knows, too." Finally, I convinced him to let the patient go.
>
> So he went home. He sat in the van in his driveway, and his dog came and saw him. It was the first time he had seen his dog in weeks, so he had his visit with his dog. Then they went to Taco Time and he ate all this disgustingly fat, spicy food, and threw it right up because his system couldn't handle it. He died shortly after that, but he really needed to do that for whatever reasons, to say goodbye to his dog and his house.

Making a career decision is not only hard and emotionally taxing; it is important and exciting. For me nursing has turned out to be an exceptional choice even though when I made it I felt like I was about to jump into an icy alpine lake. Standing at the edge ready to jump in, I knew I wanted to, I knew I was going to, but there was that moment of doubt, that millisecond before the jump when I thought, "You're crazy to do this!" Once I was in, though, it felt great, my doubt was gone. Don't worry too much about your doubts, they are an inevitable part of life, they keep you on your toes. If you do your homework, you can make an informed decision about your career based on the data you've gathered and analyzed, remembering, of course, that your emotional reactions are part of that data. Don't go on emotions alone, but don't ignore them, either.

Going Back for Seconds: Second-Career RN

Nearly 30 percent of all RNs worked in another health care area before coming to nursing. Of these, over half already had college degrees. The average age for a nursing graduate is about thirty, but it is not uncommon to see female and male nursing students in their forties and fifties. After all, baby boomers can be nurses too!

One big advantage of second-career RNs is the experiences they bring into their nursing careers. Someone returning to school after working in another occupation is often a more enthusiastic and responsible student. They make great nurses because they have experiences in their own lives that help them understand other people. They also have experiences in a workplace that helps them to understand what it takes to be part of a team, to implement needed changes, and to handle conflict.

If you are worried about returning to school after an absence—fear not! Many have done so and succeeded beautifully. Nursing instructors I spoke with told me they often prefer the older, returning student. One professor said, "They are more mature and know what they want. They take responsibility for their learning, which is a breath of fresh air." Another said, "They bring so much to the other students and to the patients. Their experiences make them a richer person. They have understanding and tolerance. They make great nurses."

Not many people stay in the same job for their entire career anymore. In fact, in this day and age, it's not at all unusual to change jobs and even careers several times over a lifetime. The gold watch, once the ideal of a lifetime of service, is dead.

Carol McCune is a nurse who became a lawyer and then became a nurse practitioner. Why? She didn't like being a lawyer and missed nursing.

Gary Meisen-Vehrs was a chemistry teacher. Now, he is a cardiac nurse. Why? He wanted more job security and was interested in science and health care. He also wanted to travel, so he and his wife, Lynnette, who is also a nurse, moved to Norway with their two children and worked in a hospital ICU for two years. Lynnette had the hardest time with not knowing the language because she loves to talk with people and, until she learned Norwegian, was frustrated by using sign language. But eventually they learned the language, loved it, and it was a great experience for their kids. (I'll talk more about traveling nurses later on in this chapter.)

Keith Svenson was a cardiovascular technician who became a nurse. Why? He wanted more challenge, more education, and more opportunity to use science.

So, if you have already gone to college, or if you are working in another area, or if you want a new career, nursing may be for you. Do not discount nursing because you think you are too old for a change. One way I look at it is that at age forty-three, I still have at least twenty-five years left to work, so it had better be something I enjoy and that has a potential for personal and professional growth.

A note on returning to school: don't be afraid. There are people at the colleges whose job it is to help and support you. In fact, there's even a name for you—the "nontraditional student." These are students who have started college and left; who are older than eighteen or nineteen; who have previous degrees; who have jobs and families; or who have various challenges such as language differences or disabilities.

Nancy Hoffman went to nursing school when she was thirty-eight years old. She had two children, one a junior and the other a senior in high school. She had worked as a dental technician, as manager of the dental office, as a receptionist in a doctor's office, and finally as a medical technician in the same office. She loved working as a medical technician and everyone kept telling her, "You need to return to school." So she did. Now she is an RN working in a small hospital and is the nursing adviser at Washington State University.

I asked her why she chose nursing and she answered, "I had lived on and off in the halls of a hospital as a child. My mother had multiple sclerosis and I helped her. I was used to the environment and I loved the work."

It is common for people to be drawn to nursing as a result of their personal experiences with illness. Often this is good, because these experiences have given you a clearer idea of what your values are, or helped you become empathetic toward others' needs. But sometimes this is not good, because your experiences motivate you to go into nursing for reasons that are not really connected to being a nurse.

For example, Robin Harper, age twenty-five, worked as a teaching assistant in a preschool and wanted a change. She thought she wanted to be a nurse because she had an aunt who was a nurse whom she respected and admired. Robin thought nursing would be a good career. When she talked to the nursing adviser at her school she said, "I like the idea of helping people. I want to do what nurses do, like giving medications, holding babies, things like that."

Robin, through no fault of her own, was basing her decision on unreal expectations, on her admiration of her aunt, and on stereotypes of nursing work. The truth is that nurses do much more than hold babies. Luckily, Robin spent a few months that summer observing a nurse in a hospital obstetrics unit. This gave her a chance to see what an OB nurse really does: making complex physical, social, and cultural assessments; monitoring and following up on potential complications; coordinating all aspects of the care of a patient and her family; communicating with all other members of the health care team; and giving spiritual or grief guidance when needed. Robin changed her view of the work, but still decided to major in nursing. She said, "It was different than I thought. It turned out the work was more complicated and difficult. It also turned out I liked it even more—just for those reasons."

Do You Have Enough Guts to Be a Good Nurse?

This is a tough question that nurses would answer in a variety of ways. The Oncology Nursing Society surveyed thousands of their members as part of an effort to improve the public image of oncology nursing. The nurses were asked to choose three words that most accurately described oncology nurses. The following is a list of the five most common words:

1. Caring
2. Compassionate
3. Knowledgeable
4. Dedicated
5. Professional

My list, not in order of priority, includes these and elaborates on what I have read, observed, and gleaned from talking to nurses in a variety of fields and their patients.

The Basics:

1. Intelligent and analytical
2. Assertive
3. Caring
4. Politically aware
5. Visionary
6. Interested in science and health
7. Appreciates diversity
8. Creative
9. Lifelong learner

Why these? Because nurses need to be the following:

1. Leaders
2. Decision makers
3. Change makers—locally and globally
4. Advocates for *all* kinds of people
5. Teachers
6. Responsible
7. Caring and kind
8. A people person

In the past, the concept of the ideal nurse might have been: someone who is well groomed, has their nursing license up to date, tests negative for tuberculosis, has no back problems, will work any shift any time, doesn't care what unit they are assigned to, doesn't care how much they are paid, is quiet, and does the work of two to three people.

A more up-to-date and realistic example is: a smart person who can think for her- or himself, wants to promote the health of all people (not just certain people like nonalcoholics, nonsmokers, or certain ethnic groups), initiates and leads the way to needed changes, works hard, cares for patients and for self (no martyrs allowed).

I asked nursing instructors from Washington State University and from Gonzaga University what they wanted to see in nurses. Most named the ability to take on leadership roles as their number one most desired quality. In other words, it is absolutely vital that you consider nursing as a profession that needs assertive, thinking, committed people. We do not want nurses who just want a pleasant or totally task-oriented job. Why? Because, for one thing, with changes in health care RNs need to be on top of the political issues that affect our patients. RNs must be leaders in making sure not only that patient care is safe but that it gets the results or outcomes we want.

The National League for Nursing suggests you ask yourself the following questions to see if you have what it takes to be a nurse:
1. Are you an independent, creative person?
2. Can you think problems through logically?
3. Do you find satisfaction in helping other people?
4. Do you like math and science? Have you gotten good grades in basic math and science courses?
5. Can you express yourself effectively in speech and in writing?
6. Are you intrigued by machines and have an interest in how they work?
7. Do you work well with your hands?
8. Do you work well in emergency situations? Do you have common sense?
9. Do you meet new people easily? Do your friends say you're a warm, friendly person? Do you prefer working around others rather than alone?

My ideal nurse is also politically active and belongs to the American Nurses Association (ANA). He or she would be well read, interested in a wide variety of subjects like music, movies, and art, and living a healthy lifestyle by eating a healthy diet and exercising. In short, this nurse would practice the lifestyle that she or he preached.

Reading all this, you might be thinking, "This is impossible, I might as well give up now. I could never be this ideal person." You know what? You might be that person right now. Or, if you are like me, you have these goals and values in your life and you work on attaining them as you go. The key is this: if you have a strong interest in simply having these qualities, you are already on your way to being a nurse.

In summary, realize that unless you have done a lot of talking to and watching nurses on the job, you don't know what they do, because so much of nursing takes place behind the scenes (the decisions, the thinking, even the caring, is often unseen by the casual observer). So, before you decide on nursing as a career, you must find out what a nurse does by watching one at work. Then check the lists above to see if you qualify. Finally, talk to a nursing adviser at the school you wish to attend for more details.

The Daily Grind: Where Do Nurses Work and What Do They Do There?

Approximately two-thirds of all working RNs work in hospitals. Most of these nurses work directly in patient care, with 40 percent on medical or surgical units. About 18 percent work in intensive or critical care units. Over 8 percent work in the operating room and 7 percent in emergency rooms.

Another 13 percent of RNs work in community or public health settings. These include health departments, visiting nurses services, home health agencies, and other nonhospital areas such substance abuse facilities.

Almost 8.5 percent of RNs work in ambulatory care: doctors' offices, nursing clinics, health maintenance organizations, and mixed professional practices.

Eight percent of RNs work in nursing homes or long-term care facilities. Of the rest, 2 percent work in nursing education, 2.7 percent in student health, 1 percent in occupational health, and 3 percent in other areas such as state boards of nursing, health planning agencies, and correctional facilities.

To give you an idea of what nurses are doing in their various work sites, RNs I interviewed shared stories that they felt represented important, or significant, moments in their careers. Not always pleasant, their stories give you insight into the thoughts, feelings, and values that are important to these nurses while they are on the job.

Crying into the Dish Towel

Sharon Reynolds, now a graduate student working on her nurse practitioner degree, mountain-climbs, ice-skates, and is full to the brim with fun, energy, and a wide range of interests. She has been a nurse for seventeen years. She responded to the question "What was a very memorable or important event in your nursing career?" with the following story:

Shortly after graduation, I was about twenty-five, I killed time working in a nursing home for nine months, and then I moved back home to my rural area. My dream had always been to work in obstetrics.

I worked at a thirty-five-bed rural hospital, where we had one labor room with two beds and an old-fashioned delivery room. We didn't have a birthing room. I got a call one night. "Sharon, we have a patient here for you, but she's not in labor." So I went in to work.

The patient was a young Caucasian prime [first pregnancy] that had come in thinking she was in labor. This is real typical for primes. Another nurse, Terry, had already done Leopold's maneuvers and couldn't identify the presenting part of the baby. Terry called the intern, and believe me, Terry with all her vast experience would know more than the intern. But the intern couldn't figure it out, either.

So they took the woman to X ray, because we didn't have ultrasound then, and, well . . . there was no head. They took another X ray. There was no head. They had a completely unexpected anencephalic baby at term, in a so-called low-risk pregnancy. The reason I was called in was to give emotional support and care.

So I walked in. The physician was a young family practice doctor. He was devastated that he had missed this problem. And the family was devastated. I mean everyone was devastated. I still remember walking into this maelstrom of people and the woman's father, the baby's grandfather, was intoxicated. He was being verbally abusive to the physician. I'll never forget, he was saying, "You should have known, you should have known." And I walked into this, literally to sit by the bed and help, because that was one of the strengths of this rural hospital, we didn't have the birthing rooms, and we didn't have the plush carpeting, but we had good one-to-one patient labor support.

I was a very new, young nurse and I am dealing with all the psychosocial needs of this family that's just been absolutely devastated. And at one point the physician offered to take me off the case, because he said that we could have one of the nurses with more experience do it. I said, "No, it's okay." So, to make a long story short, inducing this labor took three days, and we were working twelve-hour shifts, and I remember that I would be with her all day, sitting at the bedside running the Pitocin to promote labor, and talking, giving back rubs, just everything. And then I'd go home and I would just sob. I still remember doing my dishes and crying into the towel. Then I would go back the next day, because consistency of care was really important, this family and I had a good rapport, I worked to make the best out of a bad situation.

So, on the third day, we got her far enough for the physician to rupture the membranes. I never saw so much amniotic fluid in my life. Gallons of it. It was just pouring over the edge of the bed, saturating the floor, you know, just pouring. And now this woman's skin over her abdomen, that has been so tight and shiny, was shrunk way down to nothing, like an elephant's skin.

She delivered and we were hoping that the baby would be born dead, and it was. It died right then, it never breathed, and I know, because I read the autopsy report later. The woman told us she didn't want to see the baby, but the husband did. We got everything cleaned up, and it was very traumatic, you know, for all of us. And so we said, "Do you still want to see the baby. It's okay if you want to. Are you ready for this?" And so we uncovered the baby from the feet up. You know, didn't completely expose the baby. And that father just about passed out. I mean he absolutely went white and started to get real wobbly, and I don't blame him, 'cause it was beyond his worst nightmares.

I asked Sharon what she thought it took to do this kind of nursing care.

I think there's almost a conscious decision about what kind of person you are going to be, what kind of nurse you are going to be. Why did I go in on this case? There's a lot of cases like this I could tell you about. It's hard for me to remember them all. You forget about them. You take it for granted, I think we do take for granted what we do.

There was this one case where a baby died and I had to do the postmortem care, and I am not one that likes to do that. But I remember doing that with love, like I would for my own baby, because this family was so devastated. I made the baby look as good as possible for them, because of course they couldn't do it.

But we would have fun, too. We would just laugh our guts out, we really, really had a lot of fun. I mean, we worked really hard, you know, and sometimes bizarre things would just happen.

Sharon's story is not meant to turn you away from nursing. As I said in Chapter 1, you don't have to like blood to be a nurse. Not all nurses work in such difficult circumstances, but in your training and your first years of nursing, you are likely to be working in many situations that involve pain as well as joy, life as well as death.

Trauma Is Nothing Compared to This

Barb Cheramy looked at me, smiled, and shook her head when I asked her to tell me a story I thought was typical for an emergency department nurse. I had asked her about working in a trauma situation, like a motor vehicle accident. She said with a great deal of authority and experience:

> But, you see, those aren't the situations where I think I'm most valuable. I consider that kind of stuff monkey work. Yes, it's a wonderful thing to go in there, and I am a master in that trauma room. I shine, you know, I do it very well and very rapidly and then I send them off to surgery. But my real nursing skill is being in a room with a woman who has been raped and knowing how to position myself in the room, where and how to sit, and to learn and understand from interview after interview that it takes twenty to sixty minutes to make her feel comfortable enough to be able to turn and make eye contact with me; eventually, to talk to me about what happened. Those are the skills that I consider most valuable. They're lifesaving skills. I make a tremendous difference in her life. I mean, she can either heal from this or she can be crippled and wounded and never heal from it for the rest of her life. People's lives are changed by the things that I do for them. And that makes me feel good.

Is My Baby Going to Die?

Molly Butler, an obstetrics nurse, told me about using both her technical critical care skills and caring skills. She finds satisfaction in caring for patients with physical and emotional needs such as the young woman and her unborn baby in this story.

> A twenty-three-year-old female presented to us with complaints of headaches, blurred vision, pitting edema, thirty-two weeks of a first pregnancy, and she's a really nice person with a nurturing and caring husband. She had gone into the doctor's office that day without any symptoms previously in her pregnancy and now she had PIH, pregnancy induced hypertension. She was flown up to us, to an unfamiliar city without her relatives, without a support system, except her husband. We took care of her for two days before we

decided to C-section her because her hypertension was so severe it was starting to affect her liver and her kidneys.

The environment in intensive care was not what she expected. People have their expectations on how they want their labor and delivery to occur, and that's basically blown out the window. Plus she's a first-time mom and she's wondering, "What's going to happen with my baby? Is my baby going to die?" And the husband's asking, "Is my wife going to die?" Hypertension causes a decreased placental flow and smaller babies—her baby was one pound six ounces. So there were a lot of variables to deal with.

She needed a lot of nurturing, caring, crisis intervention, and a lot of teaching. I told her, "We're going to take one hour at a time and see how things go." We wanted to see if she would display seizures, or signs and symptoms of nervous system involvement such as changes in her reflexes. She grew worse and now we're talking about a life-and-death situation for mom and baby. And so, under the pretense that she is going to be okay, you are hopeful, and you do show hopefulness, but with guarded optimism. We eventually stabilized her so that the C-section could be done . . . everyone was fine.

I enjoyed the challenge of this situation because I could be a nurturing, caring person and still use my critical care skills. I was able to impress upon these people, in a gentle way, the dynamics of hypertension in a life-and-death situation. And they were really great people to work with.

God's in Charge

Nurses often deal with sticky moral and ethical issues that have no right or wrong answers. When a family is forced to make a life-or-death decision about their son, Tiena Lynes shows the importance nursing care plays in helping them come to grips with and resolve deeply emotional problems.

In southern California, a patient that I'd been seeing for about six months had a physician who had managed his care for the past nine years. The physician was throwing up his hands in frustration and saying that he did not want to continue with this patient anymore. His frustration was with the family, whose expectations were different from the doctor's.

The patient was this family's thirty-one-year-old son, who had been comatose, in a vegetative state, since a gunshot wound nine years ago. The family always wanted everything and anything done for him, but the physician did not agree with this plan of care. So I was trying to help the family find another physician. I found one, the only doctor in the entire area who would take him, but only if the family would sign a No Code, which meant that they would not do any CPR on him. But to the family that meant that they didn't love their son, that they weren't caring for him.

In talking with them I understood and respected their beliefs and realized there was also a cultural difference between us. English was not their first language. We had a person on staff who spoke Spanish, so I asked her if she would come with me on a visit and talk with the family.

My goal was to get them to sign the No Code agreement. We had a conference and talked about how signing this No Code did not mean that we would stop caring for their son. We would continue to do all that we could, but it would stop short of CPR. I managed to incorporate their belief system into the whole thing, and that was the clincher. In their belief system God was in control of their son, and if God so chose to take him, then who were we to step in the way? And they could see that, which was pivotal.

That was when, even though most of the conversation was in Spanish, I could see the light come on. The mother was sitting there, she loved her dear son, she was the primary care giver, and you could see the light come on. That felt good, very good.

Working with people in crisis situations is full of rewards and challenges. Problem solving, using technical and caring skills, good communication, and careful observation are commonly used in nursing. Whether you work in a hospital or in home care, in a nursing home or in a rural clinic, these stories describe examples of the type of work you will be doing there.

Options in Nursing

In their work nurses do just about everything you can think of. They are lawyers, businesspeople, managers, teachers, scientists, politicians, executives, business owners, inventors, exercise specialists, counselors, writers, and professional speakers.

But the very heart of nursing is patient care—what is called bedside nursing, or clinical practice. It is the hands-on work of nursing, where nurse and patient interact. So, even though nurses do many different things, such as teaching in nursing schools or directing a health care agency, the goal is always the same: to improve patient care and to promote health and well-being.

When you start out in nursing school you will learn all the basics of patient care. A lot of these basics include starting intravenous lines, reading heart monitors, taking blood pressures, doing physical assessments, managing medications, coordinating patient services, and how to do patient teaching. When you get out of nursing school you'll practice the basics and then later on you can get more education, work in other areas, or stay right where you are.

The following examples are not intended to show you everything nurses do, but how wide the variety is.

Flight Nurses

Deanna Steele and Bill Harrelson both work as flight nurses. They have both been nurses for fifteen years, working in a cardiac intensive care unit for ten years prior to flight nursing. They work three twelve-hour shifts a week, and are required to have numerous certifications such as advanced cardiac life support and pediatric advanced life support. Their job offers a great deal of independence as well as what I think is breathtaking excitement. Their chief flight nurse, Peggy Clemons, told me about an urgent call to rescue a hiker who had fallen off a cliff high in the Selkirk Mountains of Idaho.

They were climbing these mountains without ropes when one of the women grabbed hold of a big rock, about the size of a twenty-seven-inch-screen TV, but the rock pulled out of the side of the mountain. She fell backwards about thirty feet with this big TV-sized rock until she hit a narrow ledge and the rock landed in her lap. One of the other climbers instantly took off, running seven miles across the mountains to make a call for help.

Luckily, when we got the call we had a helicopter that had just returned from refueling, so we were able to lift off immediately. We all happened to know the area well because of our own hiking experiences. When we got there we saw this guy signaling us with a piece of mirror. We flew around and saw a group of people huddled on a ledge. They waved at us, but there was no place to land. It was a sheer cliff. We had to do a one-skid landing where one of the helicopter's skids balances on the ground while the other one is still in the air. We didn't want to take a lot of equipment with us because we had to hike down loose steep rock with no trail. So, as we landed, we threw out the clamshell and C-collar, which was blown over the side of the mountain by a gust of wind, along with the airway pack and some IV gear, and climbed out after it. Then the pilot flew the helicopter about a quarter of a mile down to a meadow to wait for us.

It took us about fifteen minutes to reach her. She was young and very pale (transparently pale) and her eyes were closed. I thought, "She's dead." So I asked somebody, "What's her name?" One of the guys crouching next to her said, "Debbie." I carefully put my hand on her shoulder and shook her a little bit. I said, "Debbie," expecting no response at all. Suddenly her eyes opened wide. I was so startled, I jumped back and gasped. I really thought by her color that she was either dead or comatose. I was not expecting her to respond.

By luck, the C-collar had been blown down to the ledge, right by her side. We put it on her neck, I started one IV—the rest of the IV stuff was still up on the top of the hill. We had the clamshell, but we had accidentally left the straps in the helicopter. I had a roll of two-inch tape with me, so we taped her into the clamshell. I continued my assessment as we were preparing to move her. The only injuries that I could find were a taut abdomen and her pelvis was real crunchy when I did pelvic rocking. I knew there was a pelvic-abdominal injury and that she had bled a lot. She had no pulse at all. I never did feel a pulse and I couldn't get a blood pressure, but she responded to her name.

With a crushed pelvis she was in excruciating pain. Between us we carefully carried her hand over hand up this steep loose slope. At the top I started another IV. She had great veins because she was an athlete, so even though her blood pressure was so low, it was easy to start the IV.

We yelled at the pilot down in the meadow, and with the echo off the hillsides he could hear us. Again, by chance, we had a trainee, who had stayed in the helicopter, and he helped us load the patient. Usually the pilot does this, but obviously with this type of landing he was too busy flying the helicopter. We flew back to the hospital. If she hadn't been in such good physical condition before the accident she would have died and if her friend hadn't been in great enough shape to run down the mountain so quickly . . . well, she was lucky all the way around.

Home Health Care

Perhaps not as dramatic, but certainly equally important, is the work nurses like Tiena Lynes and Sheila Masteller do for the Visiting Nurses

Association. Sheila is the executive director, has a master's degree in nursing as an adult nurse practitioner, and is very respected in the community.

Tiena is a staff nurse with multiple roles. She teaches other nurses about the work of home care and she sees patients in their homes. She has been a nurse for nineteen years and she loves her work because of the independence it gives her, such as making her own decisions about patient care.

One problem these nurses face is changes in insurance coverage. Home care is vital, but in an attempt to cut overall health care costs this area is being hard hit. The problem is caused by the fact that patients are leaving hospitals much sooner than they used to. This results in more people needing home care because they are sicker when they leave the hospitals. The solution? Home care by excellent RNs, physical therapists, respiratory therapists, and home health aides. Unfortunately, getting sufficient funding from Medicare and other insurance companies can be a problem. But this is also an area where nurses have been lobbying heavily for change.

Researcher

Ora L. Strickland is an African-American woman. I highlight this fact because there are a minority of African-Americans in nursing and yet, historically and presently, they've made major contributions to nursing. Dr. Strickland received her bachelor's degree in nursing from North Carolina Agricultural and Technical State University; a master's degree from Boston University; and a doctorate in child development and family relations from the University of North Carolina.

Through the use of her research findings, which influence changes in health policies on a national and international level, she has the power to improve the health of women and children. She has researched breast cancer in African-American women and created cultural and age-sensitive guidelines for the National Institutes of Health in the largest long-term study of women ever conducted. She has studied how men respond to their wives' pregnancies and she has done groundbreaking work on the physiology of PMS. She is an example of a powerful nurse and a powerful human being who is using her intelligence and caring to solve problems for her profession and for society.

There are other nurses who do valuable research. Many of these teach in universities, or work for the government, for nonprofit foundations, for clinics, for physicians, and for themselves. International nursing organizations such as Sigma Theta Tau support nursing scholarship and research. (For more on these, see Appendix B.)

Hospital Obstetrics Nurse

Molly has worked in many areas of the hospital, including the surgical unit, intensive care unit, and now in obstetrics. She loves this work the best. She says, "I get to use all my skills here. Everything I learned in the other areas is combined here." She works with mothers, babies, and family members during tragedies and celebrations. She is widely appreciated and loved by her patients for her work with them during difficult times. One new mother, Patti Krafft, who also happens to be a nurse, told me, "Molly is the best nurse I know of. She is caring and smart."

Family Nurse Practitioner

Peggy decided to be a nurse just after she earned her bachelor's degree in geography from the University of Idaho, when she realized that she was going to have a tough time finding a job as a "mapmaker." That summer she visited a friend whose mother was a rural home care nurse in Idaho. Peggy had always wanted a job with independence and she liked the idea of living and working in the country. So she returned to school for two more years to earn a second bachelor's degree, this time in nursing. That was sixteen years ago. Since that time she's worked in emergency and cardiac care. Now, after another two years of school, she has a master's degree in nursing with certification as a family nurse practitioner.

She works with a family practice physician and two other nurse practitioners part-time. The rest of the week she continues in her job as chief flight nurse in the air ambulance service. She loves her work because she has authority, independence, and although she doesn't work in the counry right now, she will have plenty of opportunity to do so when and if she chooses.

Operating Room Anesthesia

Janelle Perez has been a nurse for "a very long time." She earned a diploma degree in nursing from a hospital nursing program (see Chapter 4) and later a bachelor's and a master's degree from a university. She is a certified registered nurse anesthetist, or a CRNA. She provides anesthesia to patients receiving open-heart surgery and she goes to the labor and delivery unit to give spinal anesthesia to women having babies.

Janelle is highly respected by the hospital staff and especially by the women having babies.

Oncology Nurse

Stefanie Hahn has been a nurse for only three years. She is twenty-three years old, has a three-year-old daughter, and is planning a wedding. She graduated from a two-year associate's degree program in nursing and went to work in a small hospital's intensive care unit. Now she's back at a university to earn a bachelor's degree in nursing. Stefanie survived her own bout with cancer, an advanced stage lymphoma, and now her goal is to work with other cancer patients.

She works part-time for a cancer clinic and plans to go full-time after she completes her degree. Stefanie is energetic, cheerful, intelligent, and creative. She is brimming with good ideas, both for her patients and for the profession of nursing. She takes time to write to her state representatives and senators about health care and nursing issues and recently she organized a successful "Cancer Survivors Day" in her community. She has a great career ahead of her.

Case Manager

Kate Benedict has worked in home health and in intensive care. Now she works for a large health maintenance organization as a case, or care resource, manager. She manages a large group of patients, whom she first sees in the hospital to assess their needs and then again after they are discharged. She is saving her organization, and health care as a whole, money. Nurses in case management are helping in major ways to decrease health care costs by following patients from illness to health and making sure that all goes smoothly along the way. There is impressive research showing that nurse case managers lower the number of patients that have to be readmitted to the hospital for infections or other complications.

This saves everyone money, not to mention, of course, the nonmoney part—the human side of things. Who wants to go back to the hospital? Isn't once enough? So Kate in her nursing practice is a money saver, a health promoter, and a humanitarian.

This list could go on and on. There are many kinds of nursing I left out. Can you think of any? What are you interested in? Does any of the above sound appealing?

Well, hang on, because you're about to get a look at the terrain ahead and a firsthand view of the rewards and problems of being a nurse. After that, in the next chapter, we will get a bit more practical and take a good look at schools, licensing, and finding jobs.

Cool, Clear, and Toxin Free: Nursing's Rewards

Nursing is by no means a boring profession, and there is work to do at every level. One level involves keeping the profession healthy by being active in professional associations like the American Nurses Association. This work promotes nursing as well as all kinds of health care issues, from child health to gun control, to AIDS. Another level is direct patient care such as that done by a critical care nurse in a hospital who might care for someone with gunshot wounds, life-threatening tuberculosis, sudden cardiac death, or for an HIV-positive drug addict. Nurses do it all. I think nurses have it all as well. In other words, the rewards of being a nurse are many and diverse, including helping others live more healthful lives.

A few examples of the rewards are:

Job Security

This is a big reason people go into nursing. Job security isn't exactly what it was a few years ago, but there are still plenty of jobs for nurses. The National League for Nursing says that 66 percent of nursing school graduates have a job lined up at the time of graduation, the rest in less than four months.

What's changing is where you'll find that job. You may get your first job in a nursing home or other nonhospital setting. If you are really interested in working in a hospital, but don't get a job right away, get a few years' experience under your belt, then you'll be more qualified and likely to get the job you want.

Travel

Nurses can and do work anywhere in the world. You can move to places like Kenya, Paris, Australia, or Denver, Colorado. There are many traveling nurse organizations, such as TravCorps, Cross Country Staffing, and American Mobile Nurses, that employ nurses and send them around the world (see Web sites in Appendix A). If you work in a foreign country, you won't need to know another language, but unless you work in an American or military hospital, it can help. Gary and Lynnette, who worked in a Norwegian intensive care unit, were hired and worked for two years there with no previous knowledge of the language.

Money

As I said, the average salary for a nurse these days is over $40,000 a year.

Flexibility

Need to work at night so you can go to school during the day or be home for your kids before and after school? Need to work evenings because you hate to get up early? Need to work short days, say 7 a.m. to noon? Nursing offers amazing flexibility in the hours you can work. Nurses are needed in many places twenty-four hours a day, seven days a week, holidays included, so creative staffing is encouraged to increase job satisfaction.

Many nurses work twelve-hour shifts. That's a long, tiring way to go, but how does seven to nine days off in between sound? Or work three twelve-hour shifts Friday, Saturday, and Sunday and have the rest of the week off?

Personal Reward

The nurses I interviewed felt, without a doubt, that nursing brought a great deal of value into their lives. They found nursing satisfying and rewarding, which is pretty amazing if you think about how many people you know who don't feel this way about their work. And it's a good thing, too, for both the nurse and the patient. A recent nursing study correlated job satisfaction with patient outcomes: the more satisfied nurses were on the job, the fewer complications, such as infections, occurred among the patients.

If you think about how long you will be working, job satisfaction and personal reward begin to increase in importance. The age you become eligible to receive Medicare is expected to be raised to 67 years old. Try this: 67 − (your age) = _____ = number of years left to work. If you're 18 years old that's 49 years. Twenty-five years old? That's 42 more years—my whole lifetime. Wow.

Prestige

Prestige depends on your perspective. It's like looking at a view. If you love skiing, the view of a huge mountain slope covered in luscious new powder is a dream come true that can make your mouth water. On the other hand, if you hate winter, can't tolerate cold, and hate skiing, the view makes you nauseous. Life is just like this. The way you see the view depends on what you value.

Some of the things I value are service to others, good health, science and research, and persistent inquiry. These infuse my view of nursing with fantastic reward and prestige. Take a moment to think about what you value, locally and globally, and remember the praises the World Health Organization has heaped upon nursing in its "indispensable" role in the health of nations.

Gastric Reflux: Is There a Problem?

Many of nursing's problems stem from its history. Taking care of people when they are sick has typically been thought of as women's work, and women's work (which has usually included teaching, secretarial work, and homemaking) has generally been underpaid and undervalued. For instance, nurses have always taken a back seat to doctors, whose predominantly male profession is well paid and highly valued. The good news is that nurses, recognizing these inequities, have grown tired of bemoaning low pay and low status, or worse, just putting up with it, and are working hard to gain more control over the direction in which the profession and, for that matter, health care as a whole are going.

Nurses are doing this by taking political action to effect changes in laws governing the payment of nurses for their services and by mounting public awareness campaigns to make nursing more visible, better understood, and hence more highly valued. This has been done through highlighting achievements in research, publication, public speaking, and the media.

Echo Heron, critical care nurse and author, headlined an article that appeared in *USA Today*: "Nurses Can Do Much More: They'll be the backbone of health reform, providing 80 percent of primary care, if doctors will just get out of the way." Her article drove home the point that nurses receive little credit for the work they do. Ms. Heron tells the story of working in a coronary care unit when a patient had a cardiac arrest: "Four nurses successfully resuscitated him and then stabilized him—all without the aid or advice of a physician. Four hours later, this same patient was overheard thanking the doctor for the miracle of saving his life." Ms. Heron agrees "it certainly was a miracle that the doctor had saved his life all the way from the golf course across town." Her point is that nurses frequently do the work behind the scenes while the doctor steps into the room and receives all the credit, and through her writing Ms. Heron has been bringing public attention to this inequity.

To improve the image of nurses, the American Nurses Association has spearheaded a national media campaign. RN layoffs and their subsequent replacement by less skilled, unlicensed aides or technicians has provided momentum for the campaign while at the same time, studies on patient care are beginning to confirm what nurses have feared—patients suffer when the number of RNs decreases. Hospitals with fewer RNs to patients tend to have more patient complications, which, of course, costs more money and negates any savings intended by cutting RNs in the first place.

In the political arena, battles are being fought and won by the ANA and other nursing groups. New Medicare legislation provides that nurse practitioners and clinical nurse specialists (both called advanced practice nurses) may receive direct reimbursement (85 percent of the physician fee) for services they are legally authorized to perform under state nurse practice acts. The American Medical Association (AMA) has fought all the way to prevent this legislation and, further, they insist that these nurses work only under direct physician supervision. The AMA has also passed a resolution to enable doctors to bill patients for any costs accrued above what is reimbursed by Medicare. This is currently not allowed by the Medicare program and nurses are letting the public know that they are very willing to abide by Medicare rules and accept 85 percent payment.

And this brings us to an issue that has been with nursing a long time—problems between nurses and physicians. Again, you can ask any nurse and you are sure to be given examples of being yelled at by doctors, having the phone hung up, laughed at, and even sexually harassed. I've had many such incidents and, believe me, they are not only unpleasant, they are humiliating and on a day-to-day basis can add significantly to your level of fatigue. I know from talking to nurses that this problem still exists, but that sexual harassment has decreased significantly due to legislation, increased awareness education, and the potential any employer faces of being sued for allowing abuse to be inflicted on their employees.

My worst experiences as a nurse in critical care were not with the patients, angry or grieving family members, or other staff, but with doctors. I remember taking care of an open-heart surgery patient just back from the OR and having two of the surgeons standing just outside the door of my patient's room. They leaned on the counter of the nurses' station, and talking loudly enough to make sure I could hear, said, "Isn't it great to have such a cute nurse taking care of our patient?" As they smirked, leered, and nodded, I was far too busy making sure "their" patient stabilized—that is, didn't die—to go tell them off, and besides, nurses were "supposed" to take that kind of thing.

To be fair, there are many doctors who understand the importance of a health care team where each member has an equally important role, and they are great to work with. But, to be honest, there are also many, many more who do not understand the importance of collaboration and mutual respect. Studies have shown that nurses want to have collaborative relationships with doctors but that for the most part the reverse is not true. Nurse-doctor relations constitute one of the problems in nursing that you will learn to deal with, as I've said, not as a victim, but through action. You will learn how to handle conflict, how to communicate effectively, and when to seek the help of your supervisors.

Another problem in nursing is more on a personal level. Nursing advisers will tell students that in order to become a nurse it takes more than the simple desire to want to help people. They say this because it is not uncommon for people with past health problems, their own or their family's, to want to go into nursing as a way to give something back. If you think you might fit in this category, examine your expectations and realize that while nursing is rewarding and satisfying, it requires much more than a desire to help. Nurses are not at work to hammer out their personal problems. In fact, you can hurt yourself, others, and the profession if this is your motivation.

On the other hand, your problems can be a source of understanding. A student who was paralyzed from the waist down wanted to be a nurse. She thought she would be good at understanding what other people with spinal cord injuries were going through. She understood that there were many mental and emotional adjustments (what nurses call psychosocial) that go along with a devastating injury. She was clear about her values and she understood her own problems. Her experiences have helped her develop empathy—a vital component of being a great nurse.

Nurses have a tall order for the twenty-first century, changing the health care system, but it's one that we're up to and you must be, too, if you decide to become a nurse. The problems are sky high, but so are the rewards. Nursing requires brainpower, but I think that's what we have these big brains for—to use them! It's what makes us both human and humanitarians. Making the world a better place is an admirable choice, don't you think?

• 4 •

The "5 R's":
Choosing the Right School

The "5 R's" are basic safety rules for giving medications and one of the first things you will learn in nursing school. They are: right patient, right drug, right dose, right time, right route. In this chapter we're concerned with the five levels of nursing education and how you decide which one is right for you. With a high school education you can enter three of the levels—diploma, associate's degree, or bachelor's degree—whereas the other two—master's degree and doctoral degree—require a college degree. (For further information on graduate degrees, see Chapter 7.)

Diploma of Nursing: In some parts of the country, hospital nursing programs at this level still exist whereby you can earn a diploma of nursing in three years. These programs are run by hospital boards of trustees, and most, if not all, of the training is done in their facility. Diploma schools cannot grant college credits for the classes you take, so if you think further education is a possibility, careful consideration of other options is needed. Some diploma schools affiliate with colleges in order to give you credit for at least the basic science courses and these will usually transfer to another school. Diploma school graduates generally work in the hospital setting.

Associate's Degree in Nursing: At this level you will attend community college for two years and earn an associate's degree in nursing (ADN). You will earn approximately 60 hours of college credit in liberal arts, science, and nursing. These credits will usually transfer to a university should you decide to continue or return for a bachelor's degree. ADNs work primarily in hospitals and often in home health.

Bachelor's Degree in Nursing: At this third level you'll go to a college for four years and earn a bachelor's degree in nursing (BSN). About half of the 120–140 credits you'll earn getting your BSN will be in liberal arts and science. The remainder will derive from nursing classes, including clinical practice, research, and courses related to the care of individuals, families, and populations. BSNs work in all health care settings.

All Nurses Are Not Created Equal

In each of the three undergraduate levels, once you have finished your degree program, you will be eligible to take the National Council License Examination for Registered Nursing (NCLEX). When you pass this test, you receive a nursing license giving you the legal right, under the requirements of your state's board of nursing, to practice as a registered nurse. Therefore, even though all three levels bring you to the same end, an RN license, each route is different.

How do you decide which of these options to take? Ideally, there should be just one choice, for the obvious reason that all these choices only add to the public's confusion about the nursing profession. But within the profession an argument over what's called "entry level to practice" has been going on for many years. "Entry level to practice" is simply the amount of basic nursing education, or degree requirement, you need to take the licensing exam and become a registered nurse. The American Nurses Association and other groups would like to see all RNs start out with a BSN degree. They argue that this requirement would help make nursing more professional and thereby improve its image. Why? Because a college degree is a basic requirement for other professions, such as medicine, law, and teaching. Another important argument is that students need at least four years to learn the vast amount of basic information it takes to be a nurse.

However, advocates of the ADN degree say their program makes nursing more accessible to a wider group of people: it costs less, takes less time, has less stringent admission requirements than BSN schools, and is more widely available. Both arguments have been discussed ad nauseam for years because no one can agree. Fortunately, nurses are starting to look beyond what has come to seem an unsolvable problem by focusing on what it takes to produce good nurses and how to prepare them to meet health care's changing needs. In this way, the "entry level to practice" issue may be solved.

Nursing Evolution: Survival of the Fittest?

Nursing as a profession, with a structured training program, has 137 years under its belt. Nurses were around a long time before this, but anything they learned then was learned on the job, not in school.

When Florence Nightingale returned from the Crimean War in the

1850s, she was determined to develop a training school for nurses. She believed that nurses needed specific knowledge about caring for the ill and careful instruction about moral character and the values of nursing. Around this time, most nurses were poor working women with little or no education, who did what they had to to make the best living they could, including prostitution (the designation "nurse" was not based on educational or licensing requirements, but on merely being paid to take care of the sick). Nightingale wanted to raise the status of nursing to that of a profession through structured, discipline-specific instruction and to counter the image of the nurse as illiterate and immoral by teaching students how to act orderly, ethically, and with decorum.

Nightingale achieved her goals by opening the first nurse's training school in 1860 at St. Thomas's Hospital in England. But, during her time, she was vehemently opposed by doctors, hospital managers, and even some nurses. They claimed that it was unnecessary for nurses to know anything about scientific theory, much less about the new so-called nursing theory. We know that education goes a long way toward helping people gain the power needed to change their circumstances and it is thought that this was one of the major reasons Nightingale was opposed. Those who opposed Nightingale were not interested in seeing nurses, or women, upgrade their status, much less gain power. They preferred women to exercise any power they had in the home. Women were thought to be incapable of making decisions about anything else, as common belief held that women possessed inferior intellectual and physical capabilities.

For many years after this, nursing schools were located in hospitals. Students were trained by other nurses employed by that hospital. The students learned, but they also provided free labor. They cleaned bed linens, scrubbed floors, and washed dishes in exchange for the opportunity to learn nursing skills. The students worked long, hard hours, often strictly confined to the school premises, and closely watched over by a head matron.

Those objecting to this strict training thought it unfair to make nursing students work so hard. Vigorously protesting the exploitation of the students, they were concerned that hospitals were not able to competently run both a school and their business without serious conflict of interest.

In 1909, the Rockefeller Foundation released a report recommending that nursing schools move out of the hospitals and into colleges or universities. This was a real boost for the advocates of college training. The University of Minnesota started the first university training program in 1909 and expanded that to the first BSN program in 1919.

Hospital schools continued to dominate nursing education until the

1960s, when community colleges with ADN programs gained popularity. The ADN programs were originally initiated because of a severe post-World War II nursing shortage: nurses were needed immediately. The community college programs were appealing because in just two years, instead of four, a nurse could be trained and ready to work.

The nursing profession was very much against this change, but eventually a compromise was reached whereby the new ADNs would be designated technical nurses rather than professional registered nurses. They would provide care only under the direct supervision of a professional nurse. This plan, however, never came about. Dorothy D. Camilleri, dean of the University of Illinois at Chicago School of Nursing explains:

> The technical nurse would be under the direction of the professional nurse, a matter that would require appropriate licensing arrangements to be made by each state's board of nursing. These boards of nursing never did, however, create that distinction (a political move for sure) and neither did hospitals (most likely an economic move). Consequently, we have a single license for practice, with various paths to achieve it.

Today the American Nurses Association considers the ADN not a final nursing degree, but as a step on the ladder leading to a BSN. Nevertheless, while the ANA has made its recommendations, it is up to each state to pass legislation that would change the current system. This is the only way to change the "entry level of practice" issue to reflect the original intention of the two-year degree programs and to create just one pathway to the RN degree: the BSN.

To understand nursing it is useful to remember that throughout the profession's history it has been, and will continue to be, influenced by outside events. To be a nurse, then, you must have a grasp not only of health care but of politics, social issues, and economics. Dean Camilleri put it this way:

> The influence of an interacting web of societal events on decisions about nursing would be difficult to overestimate. Starting with politics, consider the occurrence of wars and their impact on available manpower, the need for health services for civilian and military populations, and the reorganization of male and female roles. . . . These are just examples of factors that, while external to nursing, form a powerful context for influencing decisions that are made about nursing.

Which Branch Should I Swing From?

The world of health care today is complex and full of change, and experts in the field tell us to expect it to continue this way well into the twenty-first century. Nurses must be well equipped to deal with these changes and that's why it's important that you make the right decision about your education.

It is not only the number of years and the amount of information you acquire; it is also how you learn to think. You will need to know how to put together large amounts of information and make decisions using a plan of care that can, at times, spell life or death. Further, you must effectively communicate that plan, along with your rationale and results, to many different people.

With the variation in the quality of schools in our country, some high school graduates could perform this difficult task more easily than some college graduates. The bottom line, however, is that you should get the best education you can to meet the rigorous challenge of being a nurse. The decision about which type of program you will go to is very important, but, in most cases, not irrevocable. If you start in a two-year program you can always switch to a four-year one.

In the past it didn't make much difference if you had a two-year associate's degree, a three-year diploma degree, or a four-year bachelor's degree. A nursing job was a nursing job. Most nurses started as a staff nurse in a hospital doing direct patient care. After a year or two, depending on desire and ability, they moved to positions as head nurses, nursing supervisors, or directors of nursing.

These days, as in many other professions, jobs are becoming more complex and the market has become more competitive. The old health care system is dying out and a new system is being created before our very eyes. Nurses need to know how to take care of their patients, but they must also be fluent in business, leadership, politics, management, and communication. So, while the change in health care brings rich opportunity, it also requires more knowledge and flexibility than was needed in the past. Protecting the quality of patient care and promoting health within this new system is the enormous task nurses have before them.

What does this mean for you as a potential nurse trying to decide on getting an ADN or a BSN? A great deal. Nurses need a wider variety of skills than they used to. Not just the kind of skills used for starting intravenous lines and reading monitors, but skills such as leadership, the ability to gather, analyze, and judge information used in clinical decision making, and the ability to communicate with all kinds of people in all kinds of situations. Clinical expertise is extremely important, but it must be more than the ability to carry out tasks. In many cases you will find that a prospective employer is looking for a nurse with a BSN to fill these kinds of roles.

For this very reason, Diane Ulrick, a student in one of my classes, was out of the running for a job she wanted. When I first met her I asked her why she was returning to school. Quite simply she said, "To get a promotion, make more money, and take on a new challenge." After working twelve years in the same job she wanted to make a change. She had a special interest in patient teaching, but was finding herself so busy being the manager of her unit that she didn't have the time anymore to work directly with the patients. She saw a job posting for a nurse educator in the new diabetes clinic, but it required a BSN and she had only an ADN. Shortly after losing this opportunity she returned to school to complete her BSN degree.

Choosing the Right Path

I won't be discussing diploma programs, because they are becoming scarce. But if you are thinking about attending one, the ADN information will be most applicable for you. You can probably tell I have a bias toward the BSN degree; this is because it's a given in our society that a college degree is the basic requirement for a profession and that nurses need, now more than ever, to get as much education as they can to take action and improve their image. Be that as it may, I do know that sometimes an ADN is the way to go. Let's look in more detail at the options.

Option 1: The BSN

You will begin at a four-year college or university and get a bachelor's degree in nursing. Many colleges offer a BSN degree just as they do a BA in English or a BS in zoology. With this degree, you will be ready if you choose to go on to graduate school.

Advantages:
  1. Competitiveness
The National League for Nursing claims the market is flooded with nurses with ADNs (58.4 percent of all RNs have an ADN). Although it takes longer to get a BSN, as a new graduate you will be more competitive. Some employers will even pay a BSN a higher salary. For example, in the Veterans Administration (VA) you will hit a ceiling on the pay scale, as well as on the promotion scale, with an ADN degree. Nurses

who work for the VA often return to school to get better jobs with better pay.

2. Efficiency

With a BSN you are ready to go to graduate school. If you have any desire to become a nurse practitioner, a nurse midwife, anesthetist, educator, researcher, administrator, or other advanced practice specialist you will need graduate school.

3. Comprehensiveness

Why is this important? As a professional nurse you must have an excellent grasp of pathophysiology (diseases) and pharmacology (drugs); as well as an equally strong knowledge of psychology and sociology. The education you will receive from a general liberal arts curriculum will give you an advantage over an ADN or diploma nurse by virtue of the diversity of knowledge you will gain. Nurses work with all aspects of health, and this is why nursing is called a holistic health practice. Excellent communication skills are essential and many colleges and universities require courses in speech and debate. This is crucial for the nurse today because nurses must be prepared to stand up and advocate not only for their patients, but for the quality of health care and for the profession of nursing. As such, you must be able to speak effectively and knowledgeably on a wide range of subjects.

Option 2: The ADN

You will attend a two-year community college and get an associate's degree in nursing. Later, if you desire, you can return to school to earn your bachelor's degree and then go on to graduate school.

Advantages:

1. A community college is less expensive and takes less time to complete.

You will be out of school and ready to work sooner than if you go for a BSN degree. Getting a bachelor's degree in nursing requires not only more time but more money. (Unless you get an ADN first and later return for a BSN, in which case it will cost you more time *and* more money.) Some nursing school advisers recommend that those with tight finances, little support, or a real need to get to work as soon as possible, go to a community college.

2. Community colleges can be more user-friendly.

For many students a community college is a great way to get started with their education. This can be especially true if you've been out of school for a while or prefer a smaller school. I've found that community colleges also tend to have more diversity in age and ethnicity of students and that classes are often smaller and more personal. When I first went back to school after dropping out of high school, I went to Seattle Community College and I'm glad I did. I needed an environment that was friendly and flexible. If I had started at the University of Washington (where I did go later) and sat in a math class with five hundred premed students and one teacher, I probably would have dropped out again.

3. You can work for a while and then, if you wish, return for a BSN.

Remember, you can always start at a community college and transfer to a university later on. There are programs available for nurses with two-year degrees who want to return to school for a BSN. These programs are designed to meet the needs of returning students. They often have fewer clinical requirements and many have distant learning programs. In a distant learning program you don't have to live near the school, which is especially good if you live in a rural area. The university I work at has a program like this and I teach students living over two hundred miles away in the San Juan Islands, Montana, and Idaho. They come to campus three times during a semester; the rest of the time they take the classes by video and talk to me via e-mail or telephone.

Three New Nurses Make Their Way Out of the Primordial Soup

The creation of a nurse is an interesting event. For a closer look at situations you might find yourself in that would influence your choice of ADN over BSN, I found three volunteers to share their early stories of becoming nurses.

"I Didn't Know I Wanted to Be a Nurse"

I work in cardiac rehabilitation with a nurse, Mary Miller, who lived in North Carolina and had a university degree in music. After several years of barely scratching out a living giving music lessons and playing in a band, she grew weary of not making much money.

One summer she happened to go to an area of Appalachia to help set up a music program for the community. What she saw there shocked her. She was not prepared for the rampant poverty and poor health. She said, "Here I was trying to set up a music program when these people didn't even have enough to eat. I knew that music was an important part of a good life, but it doesn't feed children or provide prenatal care to pregnant women."

After that Mary decided to go back to school to get a degree in nursing. This way, she could earn more money and provide a needed service. She went to evening classes for one year to pick up the science prerequisites she needed for admission to nursing school and then returned to the university where she had earned her degree in music. In two more years she had her BSN. (Many universities offer this option as long as you meet the prerequisites for admission to their nursing program.)

Today Mary is a cardiac nurse and a musician. She plays music as a life-enriching activity and she works as a nurse to earn money and serve humanity.

Mary's situation shows that if you already have a bachelor's degree in another area, but have recently decided you want to be a nurse, you can go back to college and get a BSN as a second degree. Later, if you wish, you can go on to get a master's degree in nursing.

"I Can't Move to a University"

I was discussing the "entry level to practice" issue, or BSN versus ADN problem, with Judy Meyers, a nurse I had worked with in the intensive coronary care unit. Judy told me that she wouldn't be where she was today if there hadn't been an ADN program where she lived (namely, one of those places without a university).

She knew she wanted to be a nurse, but at the time she didn't have the option of going away to school, because she couldn't afford it. She enrolled in a local ADN program, got her degree, and worked in a small community hospital for several years. Then she moved to a larger city, where she returned to school for her BSN while working in the cardiac intensive care unit of a large hospital. Eventually, she went on for her master's degree, just because she loved school so much, and got a job teaching nursing students while she worked on her PhD. If Judy had not had the opportunity to attend an ADN program, and consequently had never become a nurse, it would have been a serious loss for the nursing profession. She is one of the most caring nurses I know, she is great with her students and with her patients, and she projects the kind of intelligence and professionalism that makes her a credit to nursing.

If there are no colleges where you live that offer BSN degrees, and you want to be a nurse, check with a local librarian for information from neighboring schools. Some may have distant learning programs. These are usually for ADNs going on for a BSN, or for graduate students, but check anyway so you know what is available.

"I'm Divorced and I Have to Get a Job Now!"

Fourteen years ago Jerry Long was in the middle of getting a divorce. His wife had been working full-time while he stayed home taking care of their kids. At the time of the divorce he was thirty years old, broke, had two children ages two and four to care for, and it had been three years since he had held a job. Jerry needed to work, but he wanted a job that would pay above minimum wage and have opportunities for advancement. He would have liked to go to a university, but he couldn't afford to spend the time or the money. So he enrolled in a community college and earned his ADN. After working in a community hospital for two years as a staff nurse, he was promoted to a managerial position in the emergency department.

Today, Jerry is back in school becoming a nurse anesthetist. "If I had not gone to the community college," he says, "I would never be where I am today."

If you need a job as soon as possible and waiting to get into school, much less having it take four years, is not an option, an ADN program can be a stepping-stone to getting a BSN later, when your circumstances allow.

BSN or ADN: Where You Might Be Working

The National League for Nursing claims that new ADNs are most likely to find work in structured care settings such as hospitals and nursing homes. New BSN graduates, according to the American Association of Colleges of Nursing, should be prepared to work in all settings, including community and public health and ambulatory settings such as clinics.

The most recent statistics show that 78 percent of ADNs work in hospitals compared with 88.8 percent of BSNs. Nursing homes have 14.4 percent of the ADNs on their workforce with only 5.2 percent of the BSNs. Community or public health is where 5.1 percent of ADNs and 4.6 percent of BSNs are working. While nursing organizations are telling us that BSNs are more likely than ADNs to work outside of the hospital, the statistics show that this is not currently the case.

One way to look at it is in terms of the changes in health care. For example, fewer new graduate nurses will be going to work in hospitals; more will be working in settings like community health. Because BSNs

An Outline of the ADN and BSN Programs

The Associate's Degree Program

Where: Community and junior colleges.

How long: Two years of full-time study, about 60 credits.

Prerequisites: High school or equivalent degree. Grade point averages for admission vary.

Basic courses: Approximately a third of the classes are general education classes. The rest are biological and social sciences.

Nursing courses: Adult and child health, legal and ethical issues, psychiatric and mental health, and professional practice.

The Bachelor's Degree Program

Where: College or university.

How long: Four years of full-time study, about 120 credits.

Prerequisites: High school or equivalent degree. Grade point averages vary 2.5 to 3.0 (see the section on applications in Chapter 5).

Basic courses: Approximately a third of the classes are general education classes. The rest are biological and social sciences.

Nursing courses: Same as ADN, in addition to community and public health, management, research and statistics, and leadership.

have a broader training in more areas than the ADNs, many employers in these nonhospital settings will prefer a BSN over an ADN. Therefore, the statistics of employment area by degree program will change as new classes of graduates join the workforce and as hospitals continue to downsize.

You've probably heard of downsizing, a phenomenon occurring in many large businesses as they attempt to save money. Downsizing also occurs as a result of mergers and acquisitions. It is not uncommon to read newspaper headlines about hospitals and other health care organizations joining forces with each other, the idea being that one big organization costs less to run than a lot of little ones.

Taking It One Step at a Time

The nursing adviser at Washington State University told me that she looks at nursing education as occurring in steps. The BSN is the preferred degree, but you can start with an ADN and work from there. The master's degree and doctoral degree come next. With each step you add flexibility, the ability to get more interesting jobs, and the opportunity to become an entrepreneur with your own business.

Just about every nurse I've read about or talked to recommends that, if at all possible, you get a BSN degree first. Nurses who have ADN degrees agree. Judy advises, "If you can, just go ahead and get the BSN. It will save you time later." Likewise, Jerry said, "I would have gone for my BSN right off if I had known I wanted to do anything besides work as a staff nurse. Now I want to go to anesthesia school and I need way more education."

Over the years both types of nurses can gain equivalent knowledge, but the BSN is more likely to be able to make the jump into new health care opportunities and move up the career ladder.

There are many positions in health care to be filled. But if you want to work in a more advanced role, or practice more independently, I strongly advise that you start with a four-year college BSN degree and then plan on getting a graduate degree. The National League for Nursing Center for Career Advancement (see Appendix B) offers help for those unsure which program they want to pursue; they can also help you define your career goals.

▪ 5 ▪

Invasive Procedures: Getting into School

This Won't Hurt a Bit: Math and Science

Any degree you choose, be it nursing, engineering, law, or some other field, requires you to take specific courses called prerequisites before you begin advanced courses in that major. Prerequisites for a BSN degree vary somewhat from school to school, but usually include the following: organic chemistry, inorganic chemistry, biochemistry, microbiology, biological science, anatomy, physiology, statistics, nutrition, human development. Some schools are omitting microbiology as a prerequisite for the major, but I strongly suggest that you take it if you can because with antibiotic resistance and viral diseases on the rise this content is very relevant and worth understanding. The ADN prerequisites are less stringent and are sometimes taken in the first year of the two-year program or intermixed with the nursing courses over two years. Science courses such as chemistry, statistics, and microbiology are usually not required.

At Washington State University you take all the prerequisites in the first and second years and the nursing courses in the third and fourth years. Other schools integrate the courses over the four years.

If you are returning to school with previous college credits, you will want to have them evaluated for transfer credit. For instance, if you took a chemistry class at another school, your new school will let you know if they will count that class for your chemistry requirement. Some schools will not accept transfer credit for classes taken more than five to ten years ago. This, too, varies widely from school to school.

If you want to attend a BSN program like the one at Washington State University, you have to take these prerequisites before you can be admitted to the nursing school. At other schools, you can take them while you are there. ADN students take prerequisites during their two years in community college. Those students who then wish to enter a BSN program can usually transfer many of their ADN course credits.

Many students are afraid of taking science courses. Nancy Hoffman, RN, confided that when she decided to return to school after raising her two children, the thought of taking chemistry terrified her. All she could think of was how much she had hated high school chemistry. When she returned to school the first prenursing class she took was biology. Her grade was a C. She said, "I thanked God every day for that C."

She knew that if she was to continue in school with any success she would have to find a way to get through chemistry. She explained, "Chemistry was like traveling to a foreign land with a foreign language. I couldn't understand any of it." So she went to her school's learning center and found herself a tutor who was a graduate student in chemistry. For the first two months of the semester she met with him after every class to review the material. Her final grade in organic chemistry? An A.

By working with the tutor, she learned how to review on her own, or with other students, and went on to receive A's in all her prerequisite nursing school classes. She advises all students who are uneasy about science courses to visit their school learning center and find out who, or what, is available to help them. She explained, "If you want to be a nurse, but are afraid of science or math, you'll have to be very determined. Don't let embarrassment keep you from asking for help."

Many people have a difficult time with math and science courses because they are afraid of them. Overcoming that fear by getting extra help may be all you need to succeed. Once you get past the fear factor you can, like Nancy, do very well.

Why Me? Why Science?

If you don't have a realistic view of what nurses do, these are questions you might be asking. For example, some students who say they love babies and just want a job working with babies, ask, "Would nursing be a way to do that?" and "Why do I need science to work with babies?" Let's look at this a little further.

Imagine you are a labor and delivery nurse and your patient has just had a baby. Both the baby and the mother have developed an infection. They are going to need an intravenous antibiotic and it is your job to give it to them. What are you going to do?

First, the intravenous will probably come premixed from the pharmacy. It will tell you what rate to run the medication at to get the correct dose of antibiotic you want. You follow the instructions, but the pharmacy made a mistake and you've just unwittingly given the baby the wrong dose, with potentially catastrophic results.

Now let's run through that example again. In nursing school you took all those math and science prerequisites and learned how to calculate dosages. Therefore, you can easily figure out how many milliliters to run the intravenous at in order to give the correct number of micrograms of antibiotic. You also know from biochemistry that a chemical reaction of the antibiotic occurs in the kidneys. So you are very careful not to give the drug incorrectly because you could cause kidney damage in either of your patients.

You receive the drug from the pharmacy and this time you check it by recalculating the equation. Noticing the mistake, you call the pharmacy and they correct it and send you another. You recheck it again and this time it is right. You give the right dose of the drug to the baby. You also think about possible side effects and what you will need to keep track of for both the mother and the baby. In the end mother and baby are happy and healthy and give you a big thank-you as they leave the hospital for home.

This example is not intended to imply that pharmacists often make mistakes. But everyone makes mistakes. Nurses make mistakes. Doctors make mistakes. And your job, along with the rest of the health care team, is to do your best to prevent them. A strong background in science and math is crucial to this end. Science is paramount in giving you the skills you need to provide safe, rational, and effective nursing care. Just as a pilot must understand aerodynamics, or why the plane stays in the air, so nurses need to understand all the things that keep people alive and healthy because people's lives are in their hands, too.

Science also teaches you how to think critically and how to observe; how to reason and how to problem-solve. Ask any nurse and she or he will tell you that they use these skills every day. You must remember, too, that nurses work with the whole person. They take care of their bodies and their minds and science teaches you about how the mind works, too.

If you deal with psychiatric problems, and almost all nurses do, no matter what area they work in, you need science to help you understand treatments and to think about things such as the effect sleep deprivation or poor nutrition might have on a patient's behavior.

The humanities are equally important. By taking psychology and sociology courses you will learn theories and principles that will guide you in working with people in all kinds of situations. This is what nurses do. They apply the knowledge learned in school, on the job, and in continuing education classes to real-life situations. If you want to do safe, high-quality work you must be well educated.

The emergency department is a good place to observe nurses using many different kinds of skills. To act and think quickly they need to understand many physiological and psychological principles. Barb, an ED nurse, told me that one day she saw a woman who had come in four or five times in one month because she kept falling down. Without a science background Barb might have told her to go home and rest.

By the time Barb saw her the woman had had three CAT scans, which are very expensive procedures, to determine the cause of her falls. Let's say you are Barb, a nurse with a good scientific background. Science, as you know, teaches you skills of observation and deduction. You find out, through questioning and reading her chart, that the woman is not dizzy and that she doesn't have any arrhythmias (heartbeat irregularities). After she has had still more inconclusive tests you wonder if there is some nonmedical cause for her falls. Then as you are helping her get dressed to go home and using your acute observation skills, you notice that she has worn the heel off her shoe, that she is trying to walk around on plastic. It turns out that she just needs a new pair of shoes to prevent her from falling down. Barb said, "Those are the things that you do as a nurse. The hospital has spent eleven thousand dollars on needless tests and all she needed was a new pair of shoes."

I've given you some relatively simple examples, and believe me, they can get much more complex, to illustrate the point that science is a necessary component of nursing. So, while a love of babies is definitely not a reason in itself to go into nursing, it can be a good place to start if you are prepared to back it up with a strong background in science.

Applying to School: For External Use Only

The application process is straightforward and your school adviser can help you get through it. You will begin applying to nursing school at least one semester before you will start. If you are still taking prerequisites at that time you may get a conditional acceptance, which means you are accepted to nursing school assuming you complete and pass your current courses. You should expect to compete with other students for admission to most nursing programs. In the fall of 1997, Washington State University had 131 applicants with room for only 60 students.

Find out what the waiting list is like for the school you want to attend. Many schools, especially universities, will look carefully at your grade point average, especially in the prerequisite courses, your ability to express yourself in writing, and the reasons you want to become a nurse.

Grade point can be a determining factor when it comes to who gets accepted to nursing school in the first round and who has to wait, or who doesn't get in at all. Some advisers say their schools require a 2.5 but that unless you have a 3.0 or higher, you are less likely to be accepted. Some say that a 3.5 or higher is pretty much the norm for admission. Your best bet is to ask the nursing schools you wish to apply to what grade point they consider to be the most competitive.

When I went to nursing school I had a 3.7 and was accepted in the first round. I did well in science, which helped my GPA a great deal. Luckily, I loved science, which was probably because I grew up in a family that was not science-oriented. My father was a librarian and my mother an English major. Books were our world. Science was for people who worked in smelly, poorly lit laboratories on sunny days or who stayed up all night drinking bad coffee in gloomy observatories while peering through a telescope.

When I took my first science class in community college I felt like a rebel, like I was blazing a new trail. Remember, I had dropped out of high school, so the last time I took science was eighth-grade biology. The first class I took was a plant identification course where I discovered in great detail the interesting anatomy of plants. Doing well in that class, I was secretly thrilled. I thought, if I can do this, why not try another one? I went on to take astronomy, chemistry, and physics. It opened up a whole new world to me. I loved studying isomers, nebulas, and black holes. The idea of an invisible world where mirror images of molecules existed intrigued me as if it was a special kind of magic.

That was the beginning of my nursing career. I liked science and it liked me, but, if you are more like Nancy, who was petrified of chemistry, take heart. With support and guidance from your school, family, or friends, you can make it. Make sure you work hard, get help, and keep your grade point up as high as possible. If you fall short of the mark, however, you could still become a nurse. You just might be on a waiting list before you are finally accepted.

How Much Will This Torture Cost?

The price of school varies depending upon where it is located, whether it is a private or public school, and if public, whether you must pay resident or nonresident tuition. The National League for Nursing reports that a bachelor's degree in nursing can cost anywhere from $3,000 to $10,000 a year; community college can cost $1,600 to $7,000 per year; and diploma programs average $3,500 per year.

These averages represent tuition only and do not include fees, books, uniforms, or living expenses. (Books can cost $400 a year alone.) In addition, many schools require application, graduation, and laboratory fees. Take time to figure out how much money you will need. Start with tuition, add fees and books, rent and food, transportation, a uniform and other special equipment, such as a stethoscope. This will give you a good idea of how much nursing school will cost.

Books are available in the reference section of most libraries to help you estimate the cost of your nursing education (see Appendix A). *Peterson's Job Opportunities in Health Care* and *The NLN Guide to Undergraduate RN Education* provide information about the cost of individual schools and about financial aid.

Someone Is Going to Pay for This!

Money is available through grants, scholarships, and loans, so be creative and check out all your options. Your school will have a financial aid officer to talk to, but they may not always know every available opportunity. You must take some of this on yourself. Contact the head of the nursing department and ask for specifics on grants, loans, and assistantships. Many community groups can help you through school. Talk to local business and professional groups. Start with the American Nurses Association and work down to your state association and your local district association. Most offer scholarships or grants (money you don't have to pay back).

The local nurses association where I live offers several $500 scholarships per year to nursing students. Numerous other nursing organizations do the same. Scholarship applications often require you to write a short essay on health care or the nursing profession, a task that many people would rather not do. But you should. Five hundred dollars may not pay for school—but every $500 helps. So seek out all your possibilities and spend the time filling out the applications.

When Peggy was in graduate school to become a family nurse practitioner, she calculated that it took her four hours to complete an application for a $500 scholarship. She received the award and figured that at $125 per hour, the application process wasn't so bad after all. She was awarded the scholarship based on her merit as a student, but the probability of her getting the award was greatly increased by the fact that few other students applied, possibly daunted by the application process itself. Take the time to search out these opportunities and, like Peggy, who was working full-time and going to school full-time, take the time to meticulously fill out the applications while thinking about the end results.

Go to your library and find a book called *Scholarships and Loans for Nursing Education* (which includes loans for specialty areas, ADN, BSN, minorities, and graduate students) or get a publication from the U.S. Department of Education called *The Student Guide to Financial Aid*, or call (800) 4-FED-AID (1-800-433-3243). One excellent and easy-to-use book is *Loans and Grants from Uncle Sam: Am I Eligible and for How Much?* This book tells you in simple language what types of loans are available, how to determine if you are eligible for them, and discusses repayment options. It also covers loans specifically for health professions. The publications are updated every one to two years and will help with all sorts of creative money sources. You can also ask the reference librarian for help, and if you feel shy, remember, that's what they're there for—to help you find the information you need. What may seem a tedious task to you is their bread and butter, perhaps even their passion.

And don't forget about the military, who offer scholarships in return for a specified amount of time in their service. Besides the Army, Navy, and Air Force, there are other branches you can join like the Public Health Services, where you usually work in an underserved area after you graduate. (Exact definitions for underserved areas vary but, in general, the term refers to geographical regions where there are not enough health care providers for the population.)

A final word about money: it is worth your while to consider all options for schooling even if you think you can't afford them; sometimes spending more will bring you greater success in your education. Although Peggy started graduate studies at a state school because it cost the least amount of money, after she completed a class or two she transferred to a private school. The private school Peggy transferred to cost more money, but to her it was worth it. She said:

> The general atmosphere among the students at the state school was extremely competitive and the faculty seemed unsupportive. I just didn't see the reason for subjecting myself to that kind of agony.
> The private school was much better. I didn't like spending all the money—it was going to cost at least $15,000, just in tuition, for the two years it took to complete my degree—but it was worth it. There was a strong sense of camaraderie among the students that really made a difference to me and helped me to get through the program. Besides, the program was more flexible for me as a working nurse.

It is always tempting to pay the least amount possible when spending money, even if quality is sacrificed. On the other hand, spending loads of money on an expensive school doesn't guarantee you'll get a better education. The University of Washington in Seattle is ranked as one of the top nursing schools in the country, yet it costs less than many other schools.

Peggy mentions flexibility (being able to take classes in the evening, on weekends, or all in only one day a week) as a factor in her decision. This is especially important if you are trying to work and go to school at the same time. The National League for Nursing says that 80 percent of all nursing students work part-time while they are attending school compared with only 15 percent of all other types of students.

Over My Dead Body and Other Areas of Special Interest

On career day, high school students can be counted on to ask, "Have you ever seen a dead body?" While this may be of interest, it is not my special interest. Nursing has many specialty areas—pediatrics, obstetrics, oncology, and cardiac (mine), to name just a few. If you already know what specialty area you want to work in and you can take time to look at different schools (if you aren't restricted to what is in your immediate area), ask questions about the professors' areas of expertise. While it is true that most nursing curriculums are similar, it is also true that each school has its own specialty. This could be in research, in obstetrics, in cardiac care, and so on. You can interview a prospective school to see if they meet your needs, in exactly the same way they interview you to see if you meet theirs. This is your education, your money, and your time, in fact it is your life. If you don't know what to specialize in (and most students don't know) there are other ways to make the decision about which school to attend. Interview past and present students (ask the school's admissions office for names and numbers if you don't know anyone). You can also go to the library and read about the school using a reference book like *State-Approved Schools of Nursing R.N.* and by asking the librarian to help you find information about what a specific school has to offer you. (See Appendix A for other helpful titles.)

Remember, you are the customer in this situation, and though some schools are very picky about whom they let in, they need you in order to stay in business. You have a right to ask them questions to find out what they are like before you sign on the dotted line on the enrollment form and give them your money. Once you have decided what type of school you will apply to, an ADN or BSN, start researching the actual schools. Find a program that's right for you academically, socially, financially, and geographically.

▪ 6 ▪

At Risk of Amnesia:
Going to School

Beginning school is a momentous time in anyone's life. (Although starting your first IV line successfully is right up there—it is a real thrill.)
Whether you are straight out of high school, continuing in college, or
returning to school after an absence, you can be absolutely sure you are
doing something of consequence. Becoming a nurse is difficult, but extremely rewarding. There is so much to learn in school, but school is
really just the beginning, because nursing is a career for those who want
to be lifelong learners.

Of course, at times during your school experience you will feel there
is too much to learn. I remember studying for tests and feeling certain
that I couldn't possibly remember one more piece of information, much
less bring it back up at test time. Or worse, standing at a patient's bedside with my instructor ready to observe me perform a procedure I had
diligently practiced the evening before, and forgetting everything; standing there, mind blank, wondering: why am I here? At times you are
bound to feel there is just too much to learn, but the funny thing is, years
later, I still remember information I learned in school and then rarely
used again, like how to assess for tactile fremitus or diaphragmatic ex-
cursion. So have faith in the power of your memory: it will surprise you.

Open Mind Is Not Leaky Mind

Australian nurse Elizabeth Kenny tells us that some minds remain open
only long enough for the truth to enter and to "pass on through by way
of a ready exit without pausing anywhere along the route." The goal in
nursing school, then, is to keep your mind open not only long enough
for new information and ideas to enter, but for you to actually soak them
up—before they run back out.

While doing research for this book, I came upon the most recent American Association of Colleges of Nursing (AACN) list of priorities for BNS nursing education. I include them here to show you what you will be keeping your mind open for and to let you see your future education through your professor's eyes, as it covers much of what you will learn in school:

1. Critical thinking
2. Ethical decision making
3. Coordination of care
4. Critical self-assessment

In addition to learning nursing's role in providing high-quality care, students should learn about the development of healthy lifestyles and how to solve problems in health care. The AACN recommends schools which include the following areas in their curriculums:

1. Chronic conditions such as cardiovascular disease, cancer, and mental illness
2. Infectious diseases, particularly HIV infection, sexually transmitted diseases, and tuberculosis
3. Acute conditions such as accidental injuries/trauma
4. Nutrition
5. Family planning
6. Maternal-infant health
7. Substance abuse prevention
8. Environmental and occupational health
9. Geriatric health
10. Prevention of family and social violence

Further areas you should look for in a nursing school's curriculum are:

1. Economics of health care, including reimbursement
2. Legal principles
3. Political and social action
4. Computers

There is much to learn, but the school you go to will also be teaching you how to understand, analyze, and incorporate that knowledge so you can use it when you become an RN.

The Bride of Frankenstein: Rearranging and Sewing Back Up

You will be a different person when you graduate as a nurse. Not because nursing school brings on some kind of mysterious personality transformation, but because you will have begun to think about things in a different way. Nurses have a special way of thinking and this is, in fact, part of what you will be learning in school.

Of course, you will learn many facts, such as the pH of blood, the signs and symptoms of various drug reactions, and so on. You will also learn many technical skills, such as how to insert nasogastric tubes, attach a heart monitor, and take a blood pressure; and spend endless hours reading about diseases, surgical procedures, psychology, family dynamics, community systems, spirituality, and ethics. But, overall, what you will really begin to learn is how to think and how to problem-solve.

When I first worked in cardiac intensive care, I was on the night shift, 11 p.m. to 7 a.m. The other nurses and I used to go to a cafe after work. We would sit around a big table watching the morning customers as they came in for their shots of espresso. Very discreetly we would notice, say, a man whose face was stiff on the left side, and think to ourselves: probably had a stroke. But, no, his left arm was all right, maybe Bell's palsy. We'd see a woman who seemed short of breath and had a round, puffy face, skin that was dry and thin, and very thin legs. She was probably on steroids for lung disease.

This kind of observation can be hard for nonnurses to understand, but it is a habit that almost all nurses develop; it becomes automatic. The thinking process learned in school and with experience on the job includes knowing how to gather clues, at times even subconsciously (often called intuition), put them together in a logical pattern, and form a hypothesis.

Of course, in the cafe, forming of hypotheses was as far as we got. In our jobs, the next step would have been to test our ideas. We'd listen to the woman's lungs, take a medication history, check her blood sugar. The man would get a neurological exam and have a health history taken. With this information a bigger picture would be formed, more hypotheses developed, tested, and evaluated. This is what you learn in nursing school. It is a complicated process and one that nurse researchers like Patricia Benner have studied for years.

Benner studies nurses while they are doing their work noting what they do and asking them why they do it. She was the first person to map out the complexity of nurses' thinking and how the complexity of that thinking was related to their level of expertise. In her model, when you graduate from nursing school, you are a novice, you have beginner's mind. So you see, nursing school is really just a start. When you are there you should study hard and use the opportunity, when it is safe to do so, to start learning how to think like a nurse.

In case I haven't painted the picture clearly, let me say that nursing school can be stressful. You may feel more pressure to learn the technical skills of nursing, like giving injections and starting IVs, than you will to learn the theories behind those skills. At school you will probably get a checklist of technical skills you will be expected to learn. It is so easy to become obsessed with checking these off, and with comparing your list with other students', that the theories and principles underlying these skills are lost.

Don't let that happen, though, because this reasoning and inquiry (which at the time may seem trivial compared with the tubes, monitors, and medications) are lifesavers. They are what differentiate an average nurse from an excellent nurse. In school you will think that you don't have time to do and learn it all. And, of course, you probably don't, but I strongly advise you to try to put the technical skills in perspective. It may seem like those skills are what nursing is all about, but trust me, and trust thousands of other nurses who would tell you the same thing, they are not. Thinking and problem solving are the foundation of nursing. If that foundation is weak, all the rest of the fancy trim will crumble into mediocrity and lost opportunity, and worst of all, you will be an unsafe nurse.

Wake Up, It's Not Over Yet: The NCLEX

When you graduate from nursing school you should definitely celebrate the occasion. It is a real milestone, and not one to be passed over lightly. However, you're not quite done—you still have to take the licensing exam so that you can call yourself a registered nurse. (See Appendix A for information on the NCLEX, including how to apply to, study for, and take the exam.)

Before you take and pass the exam your title will be graduate nurse, or GN. Many students begin their first nursing jobs as GNs and the day they receive their passing test results they celebrate legally becoming an RN. When I started my first job my nametag said "Janet Katz, RN," but until I passed the NCLEX I had to wear a piece of tape over the RN. The day I received my test results I joined several other GNs for lunch in the hospital cafeteria, where we held a "detaping" ceremony and celebration.

7

Need a Brain Transplant?
Try Graduate School

The Future Is Using Your Brain

One trend occurring in health care today involves managing the care of individual patients or groups of patients to ensure that it is efficient and consistent. This can result in fewer episodes of acute illness because managers are catching potential problems before they lead to crises. Nurses with graduate degrees (master's or doctorates) who become advanced practice nurses are well trained to provide this kind of care. Furthermore, the Division of Nursing Health Research Services Administration tells us that by the year 2000 there will be only 140,000 advanced practice RNs but there will be a need for 400,000. To become an advanced practice nurse you must get a graduate degree. For a master's degree this requires about two years of full-time study. The cost varies depending on the school. Graduate tuition is often more expensive than undergraduate tuition, but scholarships and assistantships are available (see Appendix A).

Grade points also play a bigger role in admissions. It is not unusual for a 3.0 to be the minimum requirement. Courses in graduate school are divided into two areas, core and specialty. The core courses focus on research, clinical, and leadership skills, and the specialty courses focus on the area you're majoring in. If you were becoming a family nurse practitioner you would take courses like physical assessment and many, many hours of clinical experience.

Specialty du Jour: Advanced Practice

Advanced practice nurses (APNs) are distinguished by specialty area, and work directly with patients, unlike other nurses with graduate degrees who work with patients indirectly, such as nurse administrators or educators. The four types of APNs are: nurse practitioner (which is broken down into further specialties), nurse midwife, clinical nurse specialist, and nurse anesthetist. Now, for example, let's say you want to be a nurse practitioner. You must have a master's degree in nursing from a school that grants a degree in that specialty. But before this point you will have to decide what kind of nurse practitioner you'd like to be: adult, family, women's health, mental health, pediatric, neonatal, or geriatric, to name just a few.

If you know you'd like to work in a specific area, say women's health, you'd get your master's degree from a school with a nurse practitioner program in women's health. But if you prefer something more diverse, the family nurse practitioner degree is the most general of these degrees, allowing you to work with people of all ages in many different settings.

Another example of an APN degree is in anesthesia, which also requires a master's degree from a school with a nurse anesthetist program. There are fewer of these than other APN programs and they can be very competitive, but the need for nurse anesthetists is growing and the salary is excellent.

The chart shows various specialty areas for advance practice nurses, including what they do, where they do it, and whom they work with. In light of the anticipated shortage of advanced practice nurses, obtaining your APN degree is a wise career path to consider.

Stop the Transplant: My Cranium's Too Small

When I went to graduate school I specialized in education. I probably will regret saying this, but this came about a bit by accident, and if my current employers happen to read this, let me say that it turned out to be a good accident, because I love teaching. If you are worried at this point about what you are going to do with your life, much less with what area of nursing you want to go into, that's okay, just keep an open mind.

When I first went to nursing school my goal was to go on to become a nurse practitioner. When I graduated with my BSN, I initially wanted to work in pediatrics, but there were no jobs. So I tried the neonatal intensive care unit, but during the interview I decided I wasn't too keen on the people there. Then I heard of a friend of a friend who was a nurse in cardiac care. She loved her job, she loved her manager, and they had openings on the night shift. And this is how I got into cardiac. No big deliberations, no flashes of light, no lifelong goal to work in this particular place. Just an opening, a good boss, and a few friends.

Advanced Practice Nurses	Application of Advanced Knowledge and Skills	Patient Population Served	Practice settings
Certified Nurse Midwives	Well-women health care, management of pregnancy, childbirth, antepartum, and postpartum care Health promotion	Childbearing women	Homes Hospitals Birthing centers Ambulatory care
Clinical Nurse Practitioner (Specialist)	Management of complex patient health care problems in various clinical specialty areas through direct care, consultation, research, education, and administration	Individuals with physical or psychiatric illness and disability, maternal and child health problems	Hopitals Ambulatory care Community care Home health rehabilitation
Nurse Anesthetist	Preoperative assessment, administration of anesthesia, recovery	Individuals in all age groups undergoing surgical procedures	Hospital operating rooms Ambulatory care Surgical settings
Nurse Practitioner	Management of a wide range of health problems through physical examination, diagnosis, treatment, and family/patient education and counseling Primary care and health promotion	Individuals and families Women, infants, and children Elderly adults and others	Primary care Long-term care Ambulatory and community care Hospitals

Source: American Association of Colleges of Nursing Web site, 1996.

I thought, "I'll work here for a year, and then I'll be an expert cardiac nurse. Then I'll return to school." After my first year on the job, though, I saw quite plainly that I was no expert. Not even close. During my first annual evaluation I burst into tears because I didn't get superior marks in all areas. The manager looked at me quizzically and said, "What did you expect after only one year? You've got years of learning ahead."

I dried my tears, took my wounded ego by the hand, and really applied myself to learning the job of cardiac nurse. This took about eight years, at which time I thought again about school, but I wasn't sure what I wanted to do. The nurse practitioner idea wasn't as appealing as it had been, and I thought, "Why go to graduate school and spend a lot of time and money if I don't know what I want to do?" I forgot that I never really knew what I wanted to do to begin with. Four years later, when I remembered that I never really knew, I decided to go to graduate school anyway, thinking that maybe I'd make a discovery there, maybe some lucky event would come my way.

My first year in graduate school was fine, because I took only the required core courses; no decisions about specializing were necessary. But, eventually, I had to decide. I thought about the family nurse practitioner program and, because all my friends at school were doing it, I seriously considered it. I asked myself, "Do you want a job in a clinic seeing patients, including children, all day?" The answer was a clear no, because that was not the kind of work I was most interested in. I wanted to spend more time teaching, writing, and continuing to work in cardiac rehabilitation. And I could have done these things as a nurse practitioner, but I wanted to spend my time in school focusing on my area of interest.

So what next? I had to think about what I liked most in nursing and the answer to that was teaching. I loved patient teaching. So I specialized in education. Now I teach nursing students in a university, and I teach patients in a cardiac rehabilitation program. The best of all worlds. I lucked out by allowing myself room to not know what I wanted to do.

Of course, not everyone operates the way I do, so try the following exercise to help you clarify your interests. It is similar to your pros and cons list: on a piece of paper make two columns; in column A list all the things you are interested in doing and in column B what you are definitely not interested in doing. This will help you start thinking about what you might like to do and help you begin to plan for school. Remember, though, your interests are likely to change as time goes by, so let your list be flexible and don't box yourself in.

8

The Insider's Scoop
on Job Opportunities

A high school counselor strongly advises students to avoid nursing because there are no jobs. Another encourages students to go into nursing saying it is an excellent profession right now because of many new nurse practitioner jobs. Beverly Malone, president of the American Nurses Association, rejects the doomsayer's forecasts about the difficulty of finding a job these days. She does not think, like some, that nurses are an endangered species facing a dying job market. Rather, she supports the optimist's view that nurses play a central and growing role in the future of health care. Who's right? Neither? Both?

Watch Out for That Tree!

Nursing is notorious for job market swings. For instance, when I graduated from nursing school in the early 1980s there were plenty of jobs because the economy was doing well and with new technologies and hospital services health care was booming. By the end of the 1980s, the boom peaked, hospitals were filled to capacity, and there were not enough nurses to take care of all the patients. New graduates were beginning their first nursing jobs on the day shift—usually the most coveted and most difficult shift to obtain—and, on top of that, getting sign-on cash bonuses. Now, in the late 1990s, the pendulum has swung in the other direction and many new graduates are worried about finding a job of any kind, on any shift. However, a nursing shortage is predicted for the beginning of the twenty-first century due to an aging population that will require more health-care professionals. At a time when young women have so many more career opportunities than in the past, the number of new nurses will not be adequate to replace those who are retiring.

In short, the uncertainty about nursing jobs comes down to the fact that health care economics are changing and, as a result, our way of providing care. Basically, the system that we've grown up with is transforming, but no one is sure what it will become. One driving force is money and, in an attempt to curb costs, hospitals and other health care businesses are searching for ways to cut back, or to put it in more popular terminology, to downsize. From an accountant's viewpoint, it isn't hard to see why nursing, the largest part of any hospital's budget, is a target for cutbacks. This is why making predictions is a bit uncertain, to say the least.

Hospitals began cutting RNs and adding unlicensed assistive personnel, called UAPs or aides, to their staff in the mid-1990s. UAPs, with a few weeks of training, do many nursing tasks, such as feeding patients unable to feed themselves, giving baths, changing sheets, and taking blood pressures and temperatures. In most parts of the country, RNs have been laid off, while the RNs who are still working do less direct patient care and more supervising of UAPs. Whether this is a better or more appropriate role for RNs is hotly debated. Some think it is desirable (let's give up the menial hands-on work), some that it is inevitable (let's just throw up our hands and do what we're told—we don't have power anyway), and others that it compromises the health of patients and families (let's join hands and fight for what we think is right—RNs doing direct patient care, not aides).

Whatever you think, patient care continues to become more complex. When I started in the cardiac intensive care unit in the 1980s, a patient receiving open-heart surgery stayed in the hospital for ten days. Today, it is not uncommon for them to go home in three or four days. This means that instead of having patients who by the fifth or sixth day after their operation need less intensive care, all patients need close attention all of the time. Instead of having several days to educate and arrange home care, you have minutes. And remember, the first days after surgery of any kind are usually a blur and taking in important information is a difficult, if not impossible feat.

Another reason patient care has become more complex is that patients are not admitted to the hospitals as readily as they used to be. Imelda Patterson, a cardiac nurse I work with, remembers when patients were admitted just for a "rest," as if the hospital were a hotel. Insurance companies paid the cost of any stay sanctioned by the doctor, no matter what the reason or for how long. Today, a person has to be very sick to be admitted and, on top of that, they stay a much shorter time. Altogether, this means that patients require much more skilled care.

Research is beginning to show that hospitals with the lowest ratio of

RNs to patients have the highest numbers of patient complications, re-admissions, and employee injuries. Nurse staffing levels are directly tied to safety and quality of care. I read in the *American Nurse* about an RN working in a hospital who at the end of a shift had a UAP report the results of a routine morning blood sugar check of a diabetic patient. The level was very low. When the nurse asked him why he didn't report it earlier he said, "The patient was fine. He was sleeping peacefully." Understanding that what appeared to be peaceful sleep could be loss of consciousness due to low blood sugar, the nurse ran to the room.

This is one example of how care can be jeopardized, but it is certainly not representative of all UAPs or all RNs. Some nurses report satisfaction with how care is provided, saying that the UAPs allow them time to focus on managing the overall care of a group of patients rather than just a few patients. The initiators of these changes say that is what, as RNs, they should be doing. They also tend to make the issue appear very black-and-white. Nurses who resist the use of UAPs are depicted as running fearfully from change rather than embracing an opportunity to grow, as worried only about job security, and as seeing themselves as victims of a needed change. But, as most nurses know, nothing in health care is black or white.

Nurses have always been concerned with the quality of patient care and they want to make sure that quality is not sacrificed in an attempt to save money; rather they want to ensure that quality care is given while money is saved. It is not wise to blindly embrace change (in fact, embracing anything these days is not necessarily healthy). Nurses are taught to think critically, and it is through analytical problem solving that nurses, who are seen as running in fear, are logically questioning policies which appear to be driven so obviously by money.

You can see there are no easy or predictable statements to be made about the nursing job market other than that it is going through tremendous change, and no one can say for certain what the results will be. But I can say this: if you think you are ready for a challenge with change, nursing is ready for you.

Rock and Roll Will Never Die: And Neither Will Hospital Nursing

The Bureau of Labor Statistics (BLS) and the American Hospital Association (AHA) report in no uncertain terms that hospitals in the United States are cutting RNs. The BLS predicts that by the year 2005 the number of nurses employed in hospitals will significantly decrease, but the number of nurses employed in home health and nursing homes will increase. Nursing experts predict that the number of nurses working in hospitals will fall from 60 percent to 57 percent in the next several years. It is not possible to predict exact numbers, so remember that the predictions you do hear, from high school counselors, for instance, who say, "There are no jobs in nursing," are not only guesswork but great exaggerations.

Despite occasional dire warnings about job prospects for new graduates, the National League for Nursing (NLN) statistics are hopeful. They say that the total number of jobs is not decreasing; they are just changing locations. In the past, it was expected that all new graduates would get their first job in a hospital. Hospitals were always the initial training ground and they remain an excellent place to start if you can. But new graduates today should expect to start in nursing homes and other extended care facilities. Hospitals can be choosier these days about whom they hire because there is more competition for fewer jobs, and because they often need nurses skilled in specialty areas such as obstetrics or critical care. As I said, the patients in the hospital may be fewer, but they are sicker, and they need experienced nurses.

So while fewer nurses will be working in hospitals, there will always be a need for hospital nurses.

Have I Got a Deal for You: The Job Market

You might be wondering where you will work when you get out of nursing school. Of the 60 percent of nurses now working in hospitals, 40 percent work in medical-surgical units, more than 18 percent in intensive care, over 8 percent in operating rooms, and 7 percent in emergency rooms. Nurses working outside hospitals work in community and public health; in doctor, nurse, or group clinics; nursing homes; or in roles such as nurse practitioner.

The geographical distribution of nurses is reflected in regional variations in populations and the types of health care services they need. The following will give you an idea of where most of the nurses are working in any one region.

• New England (New Hampshire, Vermont, Maine, Massachusetts, Connecticut, Rhode Island) has the fewest nurses working in hospitals and the most working in nursing homes.

• Mid-Atlantic (New Jersey, New York, Pennsylvania) has the largest portion of nurses working in student health. This area, along with the East North Central states, has the largest number of working RNs.

• East South Central (Alabama, Kentucky, Mississippi, Tennessee) has the most nurses employed in community and public health. They also have more nurses under age twenty-nine and more African-American nurses than any other region.

• Mountain (Arizona, Colorado, Idaho, Montana, Nevada, New Mexico, Utah, Wyoming) has the fewest number of working RNs but the largest portion of American Indian/Alaskan Native RNs.

• Pacific (Alaska, Hawaii, California, Oregon, Washington) has the oldest RNs (ages fifty to sixty-four) and the most RNs from non-Caucasian background, especially Asian Americans and Pacific Islanders.

Salaries vary by region, with nurses working in the Pacific earning the most and those in East South Central the least. Don't forget when looking at salaries to consider the cost of living. A $34,000 salary in Red Lodge, Montana, is worth a lot more than it is in New York City.

Several career guides, including the *Occupational Outlook Handbook*, expect employment opportunities for nurses to increase faster than the average for all other occupations. Nursing is sixth on the list of twenty occupations expected to have the largest increase in numbers employed and the U.S. Department of Labor expects this growth to continue at least until the year 2005. And, as we saw earlier, the need for nurses with advanced graduate training is expected to rise rapidly as well. Most job vacancies are appearing in inner cities and rural locations in the specialty areas of geriatrics, critical care, obstetrics, and surgical care. The greatest growth is expected to occur in home health and nursing homes, although it may not be as great as some anticipate, and outpatient centers are increasing as fewer procedures require an overnight stay in the hospital.

Reporter, nurse, and lawyer Kathleen Canavan interviewed members of the National Student Nurses' Association (NSNA) for a recent article in the *American Journal of Nursing*. Despite shifting prospects, the students felt that jobs would be available, but that they would have to work harder to find and get them. They did, however, wonder how long it would take to get a job and whether they would like the job they got. According to past NSNA president Julie McGee, RN, MN, new grads should be prepared for their first job not to be their dream job. In that respect, most nurses agree that having work experience outside of the classroom is a real plus when competing for jobs. Volunteering in a clinic, hospital, or professional organization (as mentioned in Chapter 1) can help you make a decision about becoming a nurse as well as help you find a job later on.

Overall you can see that the employment outlook is good if you choose to become a nurse. My advice is that you do some research in the region you want to work in and check out your prospects. Keep in mind that as a nurse there is also great opportunity for travel. If you decide you want to leave the nest there are plenty of places you can land a job. Traveling nursing is an excellent choice if you want to see the world, and there are several large agencies, TravCorps and Cross Country Staffing, for example, that will hire you after you have some experience under your belt (see Appendix A). I know two nurses who worked in Saudi Arabia earning tax-free salaries and free flights during their vacations; a nurse in Kenya who helped manage a hospital and a clinic; a nurse who chose to work night shifts in Hawaii so she could sleep on the beach during the day; and a nurse who worked a month in Kentucky, a month in New York City, a month in Los Angeles, and then returned home to Denver for a vacation before taking off again. Nurse practitioner Beth Rosensteil, accompanied by her husband and two school-age children, spent a year living in a remote area of Nepal, where she ran the health clinic. Beth and her family consider this experience invaluable and are currently making plans to work in Mongolia for the Peace Corps.

How Long Will It Take to Get My First Job?

The following chart shows NLN data on how long it took new graduates in 1996 to find their first job according to the type of nursing program they attended.

Program Type and Percent Employed

Time to First Job	ADN	BSN	Diploma
at graduation	62.7	65.6	63.7
less than 1 month	11	13.9	11.8
2–3 months	5	11.4	3.8
more than 4 months	3.1	11	1.7

You can see that the majority of new nurses will have a job immediately upon graduating from school, and that at least 90 percent of BSNs and close to 70 percent of ADNs will have a job within two to three months of graduation.

It's No Mystery: Finding a Job

The least likely way you're going to find a job is through classified advertising, on-site recruitment, or from a faculty member's recommendation. The NLN claims that most new nurses find their first jobs in one of three ways: (1) through prior association with an institution, (2) through their clinical site in an institution during nursing school, and (3) by word of mouth.

Prior Association with an Institution

Many new graduates, especially those who take on nursing as a second career, previously worked for the institution that eventually employs them as an RN. For instance, if you worked in a hospital as an X-ray technician and decided to go into nursing, it is likely that the same hospital will employ you as a new RN graduate.

This also holds true if you return to school for a graduate degree and are looking for your first job as an advanced practice nurse. Nancy Voorhees worked in a large hospital for many years before deciding to get her master's degree in nursing. For her graduate school research project, she developed and implemented a classification system for that hospital's cardiac care unit to help improve and speed up patient recovery and discharge. The hospital administration was so pleased with Nancy's work that they hired her back as a consultant. Encouraged, Nancy started her own business as an organizational nurse consultant. She controls her own hours, makes a good living, and loves her work.

Clinical Site During Nursing School

When you go to nursing school you'll spend a number of weeks each term learning clinical skills. These "clinicals" take place in many different locations. If you have a clinical in the hospital you may be in pediatrics, obstetrics, or on a medical-surgical unit. If your clinical is in the community you may be at a Public Health Department, the Visiting Nurses Association, the public schools, or in a clinic for low-income women and children. At any of your clinical sites you interact and work closely with other nurses and managers employed there. It is not uncommon for a student who does well in clinical to return to the site for employment.

One student I knew in Spokane wanted more than anything to be a labor and delivery nurse when she graduated. This is an area that is very popular in Spokane and jobs for new graduates rarely exist. This student did two clinical rotations, one in labor and delivery and one in postpartum care. She worked very hard and made an effort to get to know the other nurses. After her first year in nursing school she met with the manager of the unit and asked for a summer job as a nursing technician (a title used for nursing students). The manager was reluctant to hire her because she already had many requests from other students. So the student had two of her instructors, one who worked part-time in the unit, call the manager and recommend her.

She didn't get hired, but she was referred to pediatrics, where she ended up working that summer. When she graduated from school, the obstetrics manager, impressed with her work in pediatrics, hired her for a part-time position on the night shift. This story is a great example of how persistence and hard work in your clinical experiences can help you find a job.

Word of Mouth

This is how I found every job I've ever had. First of all, it helps to talk to a lot of people. The more people you know, the better this method works. How do you get to know nurses? Talk to the nurses at your clinical sites; go to conferences; join professional organizations and associations; volunteer for committees and community services like blood drives, free blood pressure screenings, and aid stations at triathlons, marathons, fun runs, and other community events. To find out about professional events, call your district, state, or specialty nurses association or your local nursing school.

Read the paper to get a feel for where the jobs are located and what kind of requirements they have. For example, some jobs require certain certifications. Some of these, like advanced cardiac life support (ACLS) or CPR instructor, can be earned before you are an experienced nurse. Once you've discovered where the jobs are or what you would like to do, start working toward that goal by getting to know people and by keeping your eyes and ears open for opportunities.

I am a firm believer in this method because most nurses I know did not get their first job by applying to a personnel office, but by talking to other nurses, especially the nurse managers. They decided where they wanted to work, called the nurse manager, and set up an appointment to talk. You can arrange these meetings while still in school to gather information about what managers are looking for in an employee. Some good questions to ask are: What does it take to be an RN in that area? Are there things you can be doing to prepare for a job there? Do they hire nursing students during the summers? Do they hire new graduates? This is an effective way to develop relationships and to stay in contact with the people who have the most power to influence your eventual employment.

GI Janes or Joes: The Military

From the Crusades of the Middle Ages to Florence Nightingale making history in the Crimea, to the Korean War and the Vietnam conflict, nurses have been a vital part of the military. The Red Cross, first established in Italy and inspired by Nightingale, was later started in the United States by nurse Clara Barton. It was the source of over 2,000 military nurses who served in the Civil War (including author Louisa May Alcott). In 1901, the government formed the Army Nurse Corps to meet the military's growing need for nurses.

To this day the military trains and employs nurses in peacetime and in war. If you are interested in serving in the military I strongly urge you to explore this option. The military can help you with school expenses and employ you as an officer after you graduate. There is also ample opportunity to advance in rank and have your tuition to graduate school paid for as well.

I never considered this option because I never regarded myself as the military type. Perhaps I never gave it a fair chance, but the time commitment, military training, and tightly structured order did not appeal to me. That is not at all to say the military would not work for you, however. I know several very bright nursing students who applied and were accepted by the Army or the Navy. It was a very good opportunity for them moneywise and jobwise. For further information, contact your local recruiter or write for information (see Appendix A).

Nurse's Hats: Gone with the Wind

Nurses don't wear hats anymore—they wear many (but not literally, of course). At one time, nursing was limited to hospitals, public health clinics, and war zones. Today, nurses work in these places and many more. After graduating from nursing school, you will probably choose a specialty area such as community health, home health, obstetrics, emergency, geriatrics, medical-surgical, occupational health, operating room, pediatrics, psychiatric, or rehabilitation. These are examples of the diversity of nursing's hats, but within any one of these areas nurses also wear many different hats.

For instance, as a critical care nurse in an intensive care unit (ICU) you might take care of patients; work on a committee to develop discharge criteria; manage a UAP; instruct a newly employed RN; teach your patient's family about their loved one's illness; provide grief counseling; or coordinate care with doctors (most critical care patients have several doctors at any one time), pharmacists, and social workers. On top of all that, you may be assigned the job of writing up the work schedule for the upcoming holiday season. After work, you attend a meeting of your professional organization that includes an update on a clinical topic of interest. The next morning you may attend a board meeting of your local women and children's shelter and write a letter to your congressional representative to support legislation protecting patient safety.

It's a busy life and it isn't lived only in the hospital ICU. Nurses do many things in many settings. Picture yourself working internationally with refugees and immigrants, providing relief work in famine areas, or giving vaccinations and assisting in eye surgery for orphans in Romania. One of the biggest advantages to being a nurse is the number of opportunities. I recently attended a nursing conference where the keynote speaker, Marie Manthey, advised, "Don't go into nursing for money, power, or prestige, but for the value of helping—one human being to another." The beauty of nursing is that there are so many ways to do this, and I can't think of any other career that offers the same flexibility and rewards.

In and Out: What's New?

Health care is as rich in new opportunities as the old system was in jobs. New technologies have created a wealth of new nursing specialties such as computer information systems and genetics. Changing health care systems are greatly increasing the need for nurse practitioners, who provide primary care, and case managers, who coordinate the care for patients with complex chronic conditions. Because of health care changes nurses are also needed to evaluate and make public policy in regard to the development of new systems. The number of people, especially children, with no health care coverage is increasing and nurses are needed to help remedy this growing problem. In short, the new opportunities for nurses are in the areas of technology, health care delivery systems, and policy analysis and politics.

Technology

Genetics:

With the advent of the Human Genome Project (an international attempt to map the entire human genome by the year 2000) and the continuously improving technology used to identify genes responsible for disease, the entire field of genetics is booming. Understanding basic genetic principles is a shortfall for many nurses, so education on this topic is one area you could specialize in. Nurses also provide genetic counseling and teaching to patients, work with children and adults with genetic diseases, and do research in genetics. There is also a need for well-versed nurse ethicists, as many problems involving privacy and decision making are accompanying these new genetic discoveries. The International Society of Nurses in Genetics, a small specialty group, encourages nurses to keep up with the changes because they have an impact on nursing practice.

For example, privacy becomes an issue if genetic screening eventually allows us to predetermine whether a person is at risk for certain conditions, such as heart disease. Who has a right to know about this? Employers, insurance companies, other family members? It's possible health care insurers would refuse you coverage if they knew you were likely to develop a costly disease; employers might be reluctant to hire you if they thought that down the road you would need to take sick time; and biological family members may or may not want to know what their outlook is. Decisions about what to do with genetic information raises these kinds of legal and ethical questions, and more.

Another example is birth defect screening. Although some screening is already done routinely, the potential for more is occurring as geneticists rapidly discover gene locations for diseases such as spina bifida, cystic fibrosis, and Huntington's disease. Difficult questions arise, such as should parents be told, and if they are told, should they be advised on abortion as an option? Routine gender identification is another issue with ethical implications. If it was easy to determine the gender of the unborn child, might parents opt for abortion to control whether they have a boy or a girl?

The ANA Center for Ethics and Human Rights, directed by nurse and lawyer Colleen Scanlon, has conducted research on the management of genetic information and published a booklet called *Managing Genetic Information: Policies for US Nurses*. The booklet covers the importance of understanding genetics, guidelines for dealing with genetic information, and privacy issues. The ANA is currently active in lobbying for federal legislation that protects genetic privacy and confidentiality.

Information Sciences (Informatics):

It is no news to anyone that we are living in the information age. We are surrounded by an abundant and overwhelming amount of information coming from places like the Internet, but it is largely disorganized. Thus there are numerous opportunities for nurses in not only organizing information but in making it accessible, meaningful, and relevant to the user. Designing computer systems requires advanced computer skills and knowledge of nursing and health care. Nurses interested in technical fields should take elective, or graduate, courses in computer and information science.

Health Care Delivery Systems

Advanced Practice Nurses (APNs):

Advanced practice nurses (nurse practitioners, nurse midwives, clinical nurse specialists, and nurse anesthetists) are not new, but certain areas of their practice are. APNs are becoming key players in the changing health care environment, where the emphasis is on saving money. One way to save money is to keep people from getting sick and, when they do get sick, to keep them from getting sicker. Studies have shown, for example, that nurse practitioners reduce the number of patients that need to be hospitalized by providing extensive illness prevention education. Insurance companies also report an increasing demand by the public for these nurse providers.

Entrepreneur:

It is becoming more and more common to find nurses who are going out and doing it on their own—that is, becoming entrepreneurs or small business owners. Some have developed patient care products (a better fastener to secure endotracheal tubes), others hire themselves out as consultants (a nurse who delivers lactation consultation for new mothers is one example, a nurse who collects and analyzes data on the effectiveness of a certain procedure in a doctor's office is another), and still others set up their own clinic, counseling center, or health spa.

Manager of Care:

Nurses are in the perfect position to be managers of health services. They understand the needs of patients and they have vast experience working with many other members of the health care team. Essentially, nurses work as managers and coordinators of care no matter what type of job they have. To help save health care dollars, a growing interest in streamlining care through good management has arisen. Nurses who work in case management coordinate the care of a patient from hospitalization to home. They make sure patients are educated, have what they need to get well, and that services are not duplicated (a big and costly problem in the past). Other nurses manage care for populations or groups of people. For instance, overseeing the day-to-day health of people with chronic conditions such as heart failure, diabetes, or asthma has been shown to be extremely cost-effective. In this capacity you can work for a health care management organization, the public health services, a clinic, a hospital, or a home health agency.

Policy and Politics

Policy Analyst:
Health care systems need people to find solutions to numerous problems that arise in health care. Nurses, whose focus is on health and wellness and who put policy into action every day in their practice, have a great deal to contribute to health care policymaking. Most large health care organizations, government agencies, and private insurance companies employ policy analysts, so if you have a bent toward political science or problem analysis, you may find a niche here.

Cultural Diversity:
With the melting pot at a steady boil, there is tremendous need for nurses who are culturally sensitive and competent concerning diverse populations. An experienced nurse who is bilingual will always have a job, and one who can teach others about cultural diversity is a close runner-up. Everyone these days is trying to improve themselves and their organizations in this area, and as a nurse with a holistic perspective, you will be in a good position to provide these services.

■ 9 ■

Working for a Living

Some of the issues you will face as a working nurse are included in this chapter. To give you a clear picture I've included what RNs around the country are saying about being a nurse in the current political and economic climate.

What Nurses Say About Nursing

The *American Journal of Nursing* published survey results from 7,560 nurses responding to questions on how health care changes were affecting their work. The respondents were voluntary, so the results do not represent the views of all, or even a majority, of nurses, but they do provide an idea of what some nurses around the country are experiencing. The following are some of the findings:

• The greatest number of nurses who were considering leaving nursing were in Massachusetts, a state experiencing many cutbacks in RNs; the fewest were in the Pacific states. Approximately 75 percent of respondents said they planned to stay in nursing. The main reason given for wanting to leave nursing was the inability to provide adequate patient care in the current health care system.

Karen Tiberio, a nurse I recently met, is an example of this. She is the nurse manager of an oncology unit, and she told me she was thinking of quitting nursing and opening up a flower shop. When I asked why, she said she didn't like being a manager and missed patient care. I asked her why she didn't just go back to being a staff nurse and she said, "Because with the changes in staffing on the unit I couldn't do patient care anymore the way it should be done. With the addition of aides the RNs have so many more patients to oversee that there isn't time to take good care of them. I wouldn't have a real handle on each person's care."

It is a tragedy that expert nurses like Karen are thinking of leaving nursing. I wish all nurses would stay in there and fight for what they know is the right way to provide care, but I also know that many either do not feel empowered to do so or are just too tired after a day at work.

• Nurses everywhere reported a phenomenon called "speedup"—doing more in less time. Sixty-six percent said they were taking care of more patients and 59 percent that they had more responsibilities. Many reported downsizing in their hospitals in the push to save money and over half said their employers had recently closed either beds or units. But others said employers were adding services, due to a decrease in hospital patients and in an attempt to make money in new ways (such as adding home health and outpatient services).

• A majority of the nurses reported less continuity of care, saying they had less time to teach patients and their families, to comfort and talk to patients, to provide basic nursing care, or to consult with other members of the health care team.

• In reporting what nurses think about the quality of care in hospitals, the *AJN* report noted that many nurses felt very positive. However, the majority of geriatric and ICU/CCU nurses noted that patients were experiencing more complications, such as infections contracted during hospitalization and surgical wound infections. Several national reports concur with this. The Centers for Disease Control (CDC) reported that an outbreak of infections in the blood from central venous catheter infections was directly related to: "nursing staff reductions below a critical level, which made adequate catheter care difficult."

• Eighty-seven percent of nurses reported that UAPs had not improved the quality of patient care, and 55 percent said that the number of patient and family complaints had increased in the past year.

• The number of on-the-job injuries, while remaining stable in other workplaces, is on the rise in health care, which poses the question "Are the RNs' injuries linked to doing more work with a less skilled staff?"

• A published report by the American Hospital Association (AHA) predicts that the number of hospital bed closures resulting from the decrease in numbers of patients will level off by the end of the 1990s. A common interpretation by health care experts is that while hospitals will hire fewer RNs, home health agencies and outpatient clinics will be hiring more. The *AJN* says that it may be impossible to predict where nurses will be working in the future:

More health care economists agree that it's unlikely that every RN job lost in the hospital sector will be replaced. With half of all RNs in the U.S. over age 40, many may find making a career transition a difficult and painful process. For new entrants into nursing, the uncertainty has left many wondering where—if at all—they fit in. . . . Given what we know, nurses everywhere have every right to feel anxious about their jobs.

The survey results can be discouraging, but to me they signal the need for a new direction. Nurses are the experts in patient care, and if they think that care is compromised, action must be taken to find a remedy. And, in the long run, that remedy will not only improve patient care; it will save money as well. Those administrators who are responsible for staffing decisions must listen carefully to what nurses say and what their research is beginning to reveal.

All nurses face uncertainty in the job market, which is why so many nursing leaders are encouraging nurses to seek graduate degrees. The health care system is becoming more complex and with it more complex jobs are evolving. Nurses with training in research, advanced sciences, and communication will have the best opportunities for career mobility and security.

Let's Make a Deal:
Collective Bargaining and Contracts

I hope the title of this section doesn't turn you off, because these three words, "collective bargaining contract," are vital to nursing and you should be prepared to work under a negotiated contract. Your state nurses association is often the bargaining agent for nurse's contracts, although sometimes nurses vote to have a traditional labor union negotiate for them instead. Workplaces have two kinds of membership: mandatory and optional. In a mandatory membership you belong to the bargaining unit as a condition of employment (called a closed shop); in an optional setup membership is a choice but, whether you are a member or not, you are covered by the contract. And therein lies the rub.

At the hospital where I worked for eleven years, over 65 percent of the nurses were optional members of the nurses association. Our contract covered everything from salary, benefits, and use of sick time to layoff procedures. The 35 percent who were not members received the same terms under the contract. It is not hard to understand how the paying members resented those who didn't pay dues but who received the same benefits. Nevertheless, labor laws allow this; at every contract negotiation we tried to get a closed shop but the administration would not agree.

So we diligently worked year-round to convince nonmembers to become members.

The purpose of collective bargaining is not only to negotiate equitable salaries and safe working conditions but also to protect patients. In 1997, the Massachusetts Nurses Association helped concerned RNs retain decision-making power concerning patient safety. Their hospital had given them a list of tasks the UAPs could perform. As patient care professionals, the RNs argued that they should have been asked about this important decision. After unsuccessful negotiations, the nurses, many of whom had never been active before, held a strike vote. Eighty-four percent felt strongly enough about the issue to support it. Consequently, the hospital revised its plan and the RNs became pivotal in determining appropriate UAP tasks.

Nurses who protest being replaced by technicians or aides are often accused of fearing change. Journalist Suzanne Gordon, during an interview on her book *Life Support*, urged nurses to tell their accusers, "We have spent a century articulating and developing the science and art of nursing and will not give this up." Gordon recommends that nurses work together (through state and national associations) to uphold their high standards for quality patient care:

If nurses can't do that in the hospital where they work because of the real fear of retribution, then they have to do it through organizations like MNA (Massachusetts Nurses Association) and ANA (American Nurses Association). I think patients are being abandoned and nursing cannot be a participant in a system that needlessly abandons patients. I think that nurses have to believe in the core of their work, and the way nurses get to know patients is through hands-on care.

Essential to working with or without a contract is the principle that all involved, administrators and nurses alike, have a common goal—excellent patient care. The Washington State Nurses Association and Sacred Heart Medical Center prefaced their contract with the following statement:

The main purpose of this Agreement is to set forth the understanding reached between parties in establishing equitable employment standards and an orderly system of employer-employee relationships.

Good communication is critical to maintaining a working relationship that fosters and supports the services you and your employer are providing. Contracts can protect you and your patients, but if you work without one, take extra care to be familiar with your Nursing Practice Act and state employment regulations. As the MNA nurses have shown, nurses who stand and speak together have considerable power.

Why Should You Join the ANA?
The Dynamic Duo: Power and Politics

A front-page *New York Times* headline reads: "As Nurses Take On Primary Care, Physicians Are Sounding Alarms." As I said earlier, the AMA is adamantly opposed to nurse practitioners working independently of doctors, even though they are practicing within the scope of their nursing licenses. The AMA is a powerful organization and a majority of doctors belong to it; unfortunately, the same is not true for nurses and the ANA. Consider this: there are at least 2.5 million nurses and about 650,000 doctors. Think how powerful nurses could be if the majority of them belonged to their professional organization.

Even though many nurses do not go into nursing with the idea that they will be politically active, most want to have some control over their practice. If nurses do not have this control, then others tell us how to do our work and we do not have control over our own profession. What is needed is a good deal of education, knowledge, and research about nursing along with a unified voice to fully control our practice. Nothing can replace research-based information and group action in creating strong support for nursing. Data presented to the public and to Congress will help RNs gain professional power and political clout. In this way nurses can work in the political arena to influence and write laws and in their own workplaces to protect their patients and practice nursing as only nurses know best how to do.

The ANA represents registered nurses in the United States. The following mission statement explains their main goals of helping nurses and patients:

The mission of the American Nurses Association is to work for the improvement of health standards and availability of health care services for all people, foster high standards for nursing, stimulate and promote the professional development of nurses, and advance their economic and general welfare.

The ANA is governed by elected member volunteers and by paid staff, many of whom are nurses. Examples of paid positions include labor relations specialist, health policy analyst, director of the Center for Ethics and Human Rights, and public relations specialist. Nurses can volunteer locally by running for office in their state or district associations.

Membership is obtained by paying annual dues that are regulated by each state association. In the state of Washington, dues vary depending on employment status, such as whether you work part-time, full-time, are retired, or if the ANA negotiates your employment contract (the ANA also serves as a collective bargaining agent for nurses). Membership benefits also cover a subscription to the *American Nurse* and the *American Journal of Nursing*. To join, call or write, and you can be put in touch with your state association, or check the Web site, nursingworld.org, for more information. (See also Appendix B.)

I often hear nurses talk about the importance of working together to make improvements in health care and in the nursing profession. The expression "united we stand, divided we fall" holds as true for nurses as for other groups. Working together nurses are much more powerful than if they go it alone; a strong ANA leads to increased power for all nurses, whether it is improving the standards of nursing care, protecting nurses' jobs, or promoting public health through immunization campaigns, patient safety legislation, or education.

· 10 ·

Survival in the Workplace

At this point you may be thinking that being a nurse is not easy, that it is not only an unrecognized but often an underrewarded profession. And you are right. It requires a challenging education, hard work, dedication, and a willingness to be politically astute, if not politically active.

You are also right if you're thinking nursing is diverse, rewarding, well-paying, offering flexible hours and the opportunity to work just about anyplace on the globe that you can imagine. And finally, nursing serves the public good. You can, if you like, greatly benefit the many who are underserved and need good nurses: minorities, women, children, elders, those who live in poverty, are war-torn or disenfranchised.

Staying Alive

While you are doing all these great things there is one basic requirement, or prescription, you must follow—you must take care of yourself. You must be getting your needs met outside the work environment, needs like nurturing your feelings of self-worth, caring for your spirit, and promoting a healthy body. Believe me, and any other nurse you talk to will tell you the same, if you do not take care of yourself you cannot take care of others. Of course, this is a broad and, in a way, idealistic statement, for there are many nurses, doctors, physical therapists, and other health care professionals who do not follow this golden rule. But my argument, if you really think about it, makes sense. Ask yourself, "How can I take care of others and teach them to take care of themselves if I don't know how to take care of myself?"

I think of it as the "care equation." If you leave yourself out of the formula, the results (quality patient care) will not be accurate. I learned this rule the hard way. When I first worked in critical care I was fascinated with the machines, the monitors, and all the exciting technical skills. I loved talking to the patients and to the families, but it was the ability to work in emergencies using all the equipment and medications that interested me the most; that was the ultimate challenge and thrill. For instance, each shift one nurse from our cardiac intensive care unit was designated to function as the house code nurse. When any other unit in the hospital had a code, that nurse would go and be in charge of CPR, medications, defibrillation, and anything else that had to be done.

It's no exaggeration to say that I lived for the day when I could be code nurse. It took me two years, but I felt at the top of my profession when I could go to another unit and use my expertise to direct others. So what happened? Over the next seven years I accomplished all this and much more, when suddenly, or so it seemed, I started feeling depressed. I would go home from work with a lump in my throat and drive to work with butterflies in my stomach. It got so bad that I had to take a three-month leave of absence (after which I went to work in a different unit) and spent most of the time allowing myself to feel all the sadness that had built up over the years and years of seeing tragedy after tragedy and dealing with conflicts with doctors and administrators (mostly doctors). I also rested up from all the overtime I did to help in short staffing situations and to make extra money.

I had "burnout," a term I'm sure you are familiar with. It is used in different ways, but here it refers to a nurse who cannot care for others anymore without harming her- or himself, because she or he has become psychologically, emotionally, or physically run-down. It occurs in many different situations and to many different kinds of people.

What I learned from this was, simply, that taking care of yourself is essential to taking care of others. For me this meant working in an area outside of critical care. I started in cardiac rehabilitation, where I spent a great deal of time teaching patients and families about heart disease and thinking how good it felt not to be in constant life-or-death situations. However, there are many other nurses who thrive in the critical care or emergency environment while being able to take good care of themselves. So the important thing is to discover what works best for you by staying attuned to your thoughts and feelings, eating a healthy diet and exercising, and talking with other nurses or friends. As a nurse you are closely involved with people in all phases of trauma and loss. It is not at all uncommon personalitywise for nurses to be rescuers, or just plain super-nurses. After all, it feels good to help people, it's very satisfying, and it can make you feel good about yourself. Certainly there is much joy in nursing, I do not mean to negate that. In fact, the job I have now is a blast most of the time, despite the sadness of disease and, occasionally, of death.

There are few other professions you can choose from that offer the same freedom to do intelligent, meaningful work that nursing does (that is, and still earn a living). Unfortunately, there are some working conditions that are not supportive of nurses and that may precipitate burn-out. If you learn to become aware of your feelings and how to deal with the stresses as they come along, you will be better off for it. If you are not aware of any specific stress, look for the following indicators that often signal emotional overload: not sleeping well, changes in your eating habits, feeling tired all the time, frequent irritability or sadness, and feelings of anxiety. Anytime you are overwhelmed by your feelings you should get help by talking to a friend, parent, or counselor (many of whom are nurses). By the way, caring for yourself needs to be practiced and the perfect place to start is when you're in nursing school!

Is Anything All Right or All Wrong?

If you tend to go through life thinking about things only in terms of black and white, or right and wrong, being a nurse is sure to change your mind. You will discover more shades of gray than you ever thought possible. Imagine taking care of someone who has an incurable disease, has had multiple surgeries resulting in a stroke, and is unable to speak or move. The cost in sheer dollars alone of caring for this person in a hospital, in an extended care facility, or even at home is extreme. But what about their quality of life? One family member may tell you, "She wanted to go peacefully, she didn't want all the machines, tubes, or life support. Just let her go." Another family member says, "You've got to do everything possible, she wanted to live. Besides, it's not right to just pull the plug." You have taken care of this patient on and off for weeks and know the suffering of both the patient and the family. The doctors have said there is little or no chance of recovery, yet insist on continuing to try high-tech treatments. What do you do? Is there a right way to proceed? Would the patient being ninety-five years old affect your thinking? What if she were five years old, or an infant? Who should get to decide and why?

Nursing is chock-full of these situations and they have led to a growing specialty in health care called ethics. Chapter 8 discussed problems connected to the growing field of ethics in genetics, but ethical concerns crop up in all areas of health care, including providing health care, how organizations are managed, how you treat your co-workers, and how they treat you. Essentially, ethics are an inescapable part of a nurse's job.

You will study health care ethics in nursing school because it is important to be clear, or as clear as you can be, about your personal values and morals, and to realize that they will change with time and experience. Educating yourself on the philosophies and methods for dealing with a variety of people and situations will help you be sensitive to others' needs as well as to your own.

Difficult People: Patients and Co-workers

Nurses deal with difficult people; they may be co-workers, patients, or a patient's family and friends. There are whole books written on how to deal with difficult people and I strongly suggest that you read a few. (See Appendix A.)

Usually, difficult people merely think or act differently than you do, or in ways that really annoy you. In nursing you will cross paths with a great number of people and there will always be ones who bother you, but to different degrees. Some are minor pains whereas others are gigantic canker sores cracking and bleeding every time you go near them. I like the way I heard a Buddhist monk explain it: people just throw the knives at you, but you must be the one to pick them up and stab yourself. In other words, examine your own motives and reactions before you label a person difficult. Generally, though, if you feel bad when you interact with someone time after time—they are the one being difficult.

I've had doctors hang up the phone on me in the middle of the night, I've had managers angry at me for not doing something the way they wanted it done, I've had patients say things to me that made the hair on the back of my neck stand up, I've seen family members come in to visit patients drunk or on drugs, and I've caught patients lighting up cigarettes with their oxygen on (a very dangerous fire hazard). One important step is coping with situations like these is to learn to recognize your biases, to get help from a co-worker if you need to talk, and if that doesn't help, to talk to your manager, continuing on up the ladder of your organization until you get results. And, don't forget, always document the problem as objectively as possible. The same applies to nursing school. You have rights—even though you are a nurse, or a nursing student. Call the National Student Nurses' Association to get a copy of their "Student's Bill of Rights." (For the NSNA see Appendix B.)

At a more dangerous level is the possibility of physical abuse from patients or co-workers. Safety in the workplace is an issue that is gaining national attention from all nursing organizations. The number of assaults and work-related injuries is on the rise. You should no more accept abusive language or action from a patient than from a physician or other co-worker. Do not let abusive behavior be brushed off, even if it means going above your immediate supervisor's head. In the end, your workplace is responsible for your safety.

This goes for sexual abuse or harassment as well. I wish the whole issue had been clearer in my early nursing days. I can't tell you the number of times various doctors and even men who were nurses made offensive comments or gave me a quick peck on the cheek. It makes my blood boil just to think of it and how helpless I felt. I kept thinking, "Oh well, this is just part of the job, nothing I can do about it." Luckily, those days are over. Become familiar with the laws on sexual harassment and employer policies, and fear not, they are stringent enough to motivate any employer to take your complaints seriously.

Change Directions or You'll End Up Where You Are Headed

This old Chinese proverb is easily applied to nursing because one advantage in being a nurse is that you can change directions without ever leaving your career; you never need to feel stuck, because there are always job alternatives. Unless, of course, you live in a completely isolated place where there is only one nursing job, you have it, and there is no way you can move. Even in a situation like that, though, there may be hope: the Internet. Start your own Web site, create a homepage of nursing advice, publish articles and information, and advertise to sell them. It is being done by others, why not you? If you hate to write, try developing a telephone counseling business, or better yet, find an unmet need in your community and develop a new nursing service.

Few of the nurses I know are doing the same thing they did, or thought they would do, when they were in nursing school. Be brave and branch out, and don't ever think it is too late for you. Many of the nurses I know who recently graduated with their master's degrees are fifty years or older. After all, that's the age of the baby boomers. America is aging, and as it does, there are more healthy, active, youthful seniors than ever. Elders are downhill-skiing and snowboarding, riding elephants in India, and biking through Nepal, so why not nursing school and a career change? Why not graduate school and an advanced degree? It's probably safer than snowboarding and just as challenging.

A Final Word from Our Sponsor: Nurse Katz

Fourteen years ago when I made my pros and cons list to see if I wanted to go to nursing school, the pros outweighed the cons. Still, I was not certain I was making the right choice and, I know now, I had little idea of what being a nurse would really be like. Fortunately, it has worked out very well for me. My final advice to you is that you become as clear as you can about what nursing is, determine whether it fits your needs, and realize that if you do decide to go to nursing school there will be many moments of doubt and frustration, but just as many of excitement and joy.

Being a registered nurse can be as much fun as a three-ring circus, as interesting as discovering the footprints of the oldest human being, as exciting as rafting down the Colorado River, as difficult as trying to answer the question "What's the meaning of life?" and as scary as having your flashlight die in the depths of the Carlsbad Caverns. All this is true—if you want to be a nurse. And that is the final challenge and the reason you picked up this book—do you want to be a nurse? I hope I've helped you answer that question.

APPENDIX A
Resources

Suggested Reading

This list of books, journal articles, and Web sites is far from comprehensive, but it will give you the insight of others besides myself. As noted, I consider *Life Support* by Suzanne Gordon at the top of the list—if you choose to read only one book, read this one. As for nursing journals, there are hundreds, so I've listed several general ones that can provide both a broader picture of nursing and a classified section to scan for jobs. The Web sites are fun to browse, and they will give you ideas of what nurses are doing in the areas of practice, research, and teaching.

Books

Life Support: Three Nurses on the Front Lines, by Suzanne Gordon. Little, Brown & Co., 1997. An investigative journalist and health care specialist, Gordon took a special interest in nursing after her personal experiences in a hospital. Following three expert RNs from Boston's Beth Israel Hospital, she provides a close-up on the profession of caring for patients and families, including nursing history, nurse-doctor relations, and complex hospital restructuring. Get this book and read it right away for the best coverage of the nursing profession in an immensely readable form.

Condition Critical: The Story of a Nurse Continues, by Echo Heron. Fawcett Columbine, 1994. *Intensive Care Nurse: The Story of a Nurse*, by Echo Heron. Ivy Books, 1987. *Tending Lives: Nurses on the Medical Front*, by Echo Heron. Ivy Books, 1998. In her books, Heron, an outspoken advocate of nursing, gives you both an insider's look at real nursing and a good read.

From Novice to Expert: Excellence and Power in Clinical Nursing Practice, by Patricia Benner. Addison-Wesley, 1984. A classic that rings as true today as the day it was written. Benner describes exactly what RNs do for their patients and offers a fascinating look at the thinking and intuition behind their actions. Required reading for many nursing courses, Benner's book provides a quintessential and inspiring definition of nursing.

Notes on Nursing: What It Is and Is Not, by Florence Nightingale. Dover Publications, 1969. Nightingale, the founder of modern nursing, gives us the original definition of the professional nurse. First published in 1859 (the same year as Darwin's *On the Origin of Species*), it is fascinating reading.

Florence Nightingale, by Cecil Woodham-Smith. Constable, 1950. For this now classic biography, Woodham-Smith was able to use important private papers previously withheld from public viewing by the Nightingale family. She tells the story of how the young Nightingale went from upper-class society to the "degrading" profession of nursing, of her estrangement from her family, and, finally, of her rise to become one of the most powerful and famous women in history.

Ordered to Care: The Dilemma of American Nursing, 1850–1945, by Susan Reverby. Cambridge University Press, 1987. Includes a history of nursing, women's issues, and working women. An excellent book to read to gain an understanding of problems faced by nurses today.

Gender and the Professional Predicament in Nursing, by Celia Davies. Open University Press, 1995. If you are interested in women's studies, health policymaking, or the meaning of nursing care, this book is for you.

Journals

*The American Nurse: The Official Publication of
the American Nurses Association*
600 Maryland Avenue SW, Suite 100 W
Washington, DC 20024
(202) 651-7000
E-mail: **TANeditor@ANA.org**
www.nursingworld.org No other publication gives you a better look quickly at what is happening in nursing. Articles cover issues of concern for nurses, actions nurses are taking to solve health care's problems, and legislative matters the ANA is lobbying for. *American Nurse* is an excel-

lent way to get the "big picture" of nursing, including a classified jobs section, information on grants, and upcoming educational offerings.

American Journal of Nursing
PO Box 50480
Boulder, CO 80322-0480
1-800-627-0484
www.nursingcenter.com The *AJN* comes by subscription or with membership in the ANA. Their Web site includes information on continuing education for nurses and a career center with work listed by geographic regions. Their annual Career Guide is also found here, with job listings for nurses by specialty area and location.

Nursing
1111 Bethlehem Pike
PO Box 908
Springhouse, PA 19477
1-800-633-2648
www.nursing98.com *Nursing98* has the largest circulation of any nursing journal and covers clinical topics such as new technologies and medications, current treatment of diseases, and other practical tips. There's also a classified advertising section which includes job listings. The Web site is chock-full of links for career advice and, best of all, for traveling nurses. You can find out what traveling nursing is all about and, under American Mobile Nursing, learn what traveling nursing is, how to choose the right company, and safety tips.

American Nurses Association Publications

To order publications call 1-800-637-0323
For information on additional ANA publications, visit their Web site, listed below.

Implementing Nursing's Report Card: A Study of RN Staffing, Length of Stay and Patient Outcomes. Publication No. Q-1. $15.00, $10.50 ANA members. The best resource for research on RN staffing levels and the quality of patient care.

What You Need to Know About Today's Workforce: A Survival Guide for Nurses. Publication No. EC-151. $25.95, $16.95 ANA members. Covers over 70 workplace topics from employee rights to conflict management.

Web Sites

There is an immense amount of information on the Internet from and for nurses, although finding it efficiently can be a problem. This list gives the important sites from which you'll find information on just about everything, including job postings, tips on interviewing and résumés, schools, the NCLEX exam, financial aid, general health, what other nurses are concerned about via chat rooms, and enough legislative information to keep you busy writing letters or e-mail to your senators and representatives.

Kaplan Educational Centers: www.kaplan.com
You can find out about business, law, medicine and nursing specialties as well as other general career information, such as résumé writing, interview skills, financial aid, college entrance exams, and graduate school. Under Nursing there is a career path with examples of types of degrees (ADN, BSN, MSN) and job opportunities for each.

National Council for International Health: www.ncih.org
If you are interested in international health, then visit this private nonprofit organization's site. It will give you information on current international health issues, opportunities for student networks (undergraduate and graduate students), and links to overseas job opportunities.

NursingNet: www.nursingnet.org
This site is oriented toward references that include employment opportunities, chat rooms, and a piece about nursing history with pictures you can download.

Nurseone Homepage: www.nurseone.com/jobs.htm
Provides links to national job search pages for nurses in the form of an index that is easy to use.

Nursing Resource Home Page: www.nursingnet.com
An all-around general nursing site with access to information on financial aid, publications, all kinds of health statistics, and career advice. Lists state boards of nursing for the United States and the provinces of Canada.

Nursing World: www.nursingworld.org
American Nurses Association Web site includes all kinds of association news, health care updates, publications and career information. Includes

international nursing opportunities, a legislative branch, state organizations, educational offerings, the *On-line Journal of Issues in Nursing* (one new topic is chosen for each issue), and ethnic and minority fellowship sources.

Sigma Theta Tau International, Honor Society of Nursing: www.stti.iupui.edu

Visit this site to find out more about nursing scholarships and research. Sigma Theta Tau holds conferences, and presents awards and grants scholarships to its members around the world. The site is also the place to find out what's needed to become inducted into the society.

The Webster: www.katsden.com/nursing/index.html

This is a fun site I recommend for an eclectic view of nursing. Pediatric nurse and site creator Kathi Webster is particularly interested in death and dying, and social and spiritual issues. What I like are all the links to rare and enticing places like the Florence Project ("nurses uniting to return health to health care") and the Tribal Voice (including chat rooms and information by Native American nurses).

Special Information and Support Resources

Multicultural and Minority Nurses

Contact any of the following groups for information and support about nursing and your area of interest or concern.

National Association of Hispanic Nurses
1501 16th Street NW
Washington, DC 20036
(202) 387-2477

National Black Nurses Association, Inc.
1511 K Street NW, Suite 415
Washington, DC 20005
(202) 393-6870

The American Assembly for Men in Nursing
7794 Grove Drive
Pensacola, FL 32514
(904) 474-0144
E-mail: aamn@aol.com

Transcultural Nursing Society
College of Nursing and Health
Madonna University
36600 Schoolcraft Road
Livonia, MI 48150
1-888-432-5470

Handling Interpersonal Issues on the Job
Coping with Difficult People
Robert K. Bramson
Dell Publishing

Learning to Listen: Positive Approaches and People with Difficult Behavior
Herman Lovett
Paul H. Brooks Publishers

How to Communicate with "Difficult People"
Anne Kimbell Relph and Karen Wilson
Enterprising Woman

Working with Difficult People
Muriel Solomon
Prentice Hall Publishers

Observing Nurses in Action

As far as I know, there is no formal setup for watching nurses on the job, but it is easy enough to do. If you don't already know a nurse, try the following sources and they can hook you up with the right person.

Local Hospital, Home Health Agency, Public Health Department. Call one of these in your area and ask to speak to either the educational services department or, if there isn't one, try the director of nursing. Explain that you are interested in nursing as a career and would like to observe an RN at work. They should be able to help you connect with one.

Local Nursing School. Call the admissions office or career placement office and tell them what you want to do (see above). Most universities or colleges with a nursing school will have a nursing adviser who will be thrilled at your request and gladly help you out.

Career

The following references cover the topics of finding work in nursing, employment outlooks according to government and nursing organizations who predict such things, and guides to help you decide on a career. Again, this list is far from comprehensive. Use it to get started, and remember, go to the library and ask the reference librarian for help.

Books

*Career Development Services (CDS) & Nurses-TravCorps**
American Association of Critical Care
1-888-AACN-JOB (222-6562)
* For members of AACN
Interested in critical care? Visit their Web site: **www.aacn.org**

Encyclopedia of Careers and Vocational Guidance. J. O. Ferguson Publishing. A frequently updated reference book which you should be able to find in the library. Lists almost every job imaginable and will help give you an idea of other work in the health care field in addition to nursing.

Healthcare Career Directory—Nurses and Physicians, Bradley J. Morgan, ed. Washington, DC: Visible Ink, 1993. Look for this in the library for advice on what to expect on the job, help in preparing résumés, tips on interviewing, and other pearls of wisdom about getting a job.

How I Became a Nurse Entrepreneur: Tales from Fifty Nurses in Business. National Nurses in Business Association, 1997. Want to start your own business? If so, this may be a good book for you. It provides real-life information on business possibilities and how fifty nurses became business owners.

Occupational Outlook Handbook. Bureau of Labor Statistics and U.S. Department of Labor. Bulletin 2470. This is another standard reference, updated regularly, with information on salaries, employment prospects, and expected growth of various occupations and professions.

Peterson's Job Opportunities in Health Care
PO Box 2123
Princeton, NJ 08543-2123
1-800-338-3282
www.petersons.com

You'll find this in any library—it's a standard career reference. It includes information on nursing and other health careers along with employer profiles. The Web site covers financial aid and professional organizations for nursing and many other fields.

Profiles of the Newly Licensed Nurse: Historical Trends and Future Implications, by D. Louden, L. Crawford, and S. Trotman. New York: National League for Nursing Publication No. 19-2700, 1996, 3rd ed. This is chock-full of interesting statistics on where, what, and how new nurses are doing.

The Pfizer Guide: Nursing Career Opportunities, Mary O. Mundinger, ed. Columbia University School of Nursing, Merritt Communications, 1994. (860) 395-0528. You should find this in any health sciences library if not in the public library. Look for updated versions every four or five years.

Schools and Financial Aid

Your primary interest at this point may be gathering information on schools and how to finance your education; if so, the resources listed below will meet your needs. There are many general college guides and I've included a few with their Web sites. Others are specific to nursing.

Nursing Schools
Order these National League for Nursing (NLN) publications by calling (212) 989-9393 or (800) 669-9656, or write:
350 Hudson Street, 4th Floor
New York, NY 10014
Many nursing school libraries will also have them, so ask the reference librarian.

State-Approved Schools of Nursing R.N. NLN Publication No. 19-686X. Lists every nursing school in the United States and some in Canada. Includes tuitions, school qualifications, and admission requirements.

NLN Guide to Undergraduate RN Education. NLN Publication No. 41-2685. Gives good information about nursing schools and applying.

Peterson's Guide to Nursing Programs: Baccalaureate and Graduate Nursing Education in the U.S., and Canada. This library reference book gives you everything you need on schools and requirements.

For more general college information try the following Web sites:

The Princeton Review, www.princetonreview.com Reported to be the best unbiased college information guide.

Peterson's Education Center, www.petersons.com/ugrad A complete college information guide.

Scholarships and Financial Aid
AmeriCorps
The Corporation for National and Community Service
1201 New York Avenue NW
Washington, DC 20525
1-800-942-2677
Provides full-time awards in return for community service work. You can work before, during, or after your college education and use the award either to pay current school expenses or to repay loans.

Loans and Grants from Uncle Sam: Am I Eligible and for How Much? by Anna J. Leider. Octameron, 1996.
I love this book! It's short and organized and therefore, to my mind, easy to use. The only disadvantage is that it covers only government loans, but that's where you will probably be looking. However, don't forget nongovernmental sources of aid (covered by other sources on this list).

National Health Service Corps
2070 Chain Bridge Road, Suite 450
Vienna, VA 22182
1-800-221-9393
www.bphc.hrsa.dhhs.gov/nhsc/nhsc.htm
May be of interest if you plan to pursue graduate education. They will pay for your tuition if you qualify and agree to work in a federally designated underserved area for an agreed-upon length of time.

Peterson's College Money Handbook. Published each year by Peterson's, it can be found in the library reference section. Contains information on 1,700 colleges and sources for financial aid.

Scholarships and Loans for Nursing Education. NLN Publication No. 41-6789. Lists many loans and scholarship opportunities you may not find elsewhere. Look for this book in a nursing school library or ask your public librarian to get it for you.

The Foundation of the National Student Nurses' Association, Inc.
555 West 57th Street
New York, NY 10019
www.nsna.org
The NSNA foundation is a good source to check for financial aid and other information about being a nursing student. Check their Web site to find all kinds of nursing student advice, the code of ethics, conference announcements, career center and chapter links, additional NCLEX review, and much more.

The 1997–98 Student Guide to Financial Aid
U.S. Department of Education
1-800-4-FED-AID (800-433-3243)
www.ed.gov/prog-info/SFA/studentguide
Standard guide used by all students seeking government loans. Explains the different types and what to do to apply for them. The 800 number gives you general information on loans and updates on specific lender information in your area.

The Complete Scholarship Book. Published by Sourcebooks. Also in the reference section of the library, this book covers college costs and where you can apply for loans, grants, and scholarships.

General college financial aid Web sites:
www.fastweb.com
www.collegeboard.org/fundfinder/bin/fundfind01.pl
www.collegeedge.com/FA

Other sources to investigate for requesting financial aid:
Community organizations such as YWCA, 4-H Club, Elks, Kiwanis, Jaycees, Chamber of Commerce, Girl or Boy Scouts, religious organizations, private foundations, your current place of employment and labor union.

Survival and Licensing Exam
Mosby's Tour Guide to Nursing School, 3rd ed., by Melodie Chenevert. Mosby, 1995. This book, written in collaboration with the National Student Nurses' Association, covers important points like determining whether you want to be a nurse, getting into school, length and cost of programs, and making it to graduation. Especially well done is the lengthy appendix on the NCLEX exam.

The Military

For information on obtaining financing through the military to cover your schooling, you can write to:

Assistant Secretary of Defense (Health Affairs)

The Pentagon

Washington, DC 20301

For further information on military programs and health services careers, look in the library for this monthly newsletter aimed at high school students and guidance counselors, or inquire via e-mail or regular mail.

Profile Newsletter

DoD High School News Service

1877 Dillingham Blvd.

Norfolk, VA 23511-3097

(804) 444-2828

E-mail: **RDODGE@FORCE.CNSL.SPEAR.NAVY.MIL**

APPENDIX B
Nursing Organizations

General Organizations

This is not meant to be a complete list of all nursing organizations. For others, visit the Internet nursing Web sites (see Appendix A).

American Nurses Association
600 Maryland Avenue SW, Suite 100 W.
Washington, DC 20024-2571
1-800-274-4262
www.nursingworld.org

American Association of Colleges of Nursing
One Dupont Circle NW, Suite 530
Washington, DC 20036
Phone: (202) 463-6930
Fax: (202) 785-8320
E-mail: **webmaster@aacn.nche.edu**

Canadian Nurses' Association
50 Driveway
Ottawa, ON
K2P 1E2 Canada
(613) 237-2133

National League for Nursing
Communications Department
350 Hudson Street, 4th Floor
New York, NY 10014
(212) 989-9393
Center for Career Advancement
1-800-669-9656 ext. 143

National Student Nurses' Association
555 West 57th Street, Suite 1325
New York, NY 10019
(212) 581-2211

Specialty Organizations

Academy of Medical-Surgical Nurses
East Holly Avenue, Box 56
Pitman, NJ 08071
(609) 256-2323

American College of Nurse Practitioners
1090 Vermont Avenue NW, Suite 80
Washington, DC 20005
(202) 408-7050
E-mail: **acnp@nurse.org**

American Academy of Ambulatory Care Nursing
Box 56, Woodbury Road
Pitman, NJ 08071
(609) 256-2350

American Academy of Nurse Practitioners
Capitol Station
LBJ Building
PO Box 12846
Austin, TX 78711
(512) 442-4262

American Association of Critical-Care Nurses
101 Columbia
Aliso Viejo, CA 92656-1491
(714) 362-2000 or 1-800-899-AACN ext. 2226
E-mail: **aacinfo@aacn.org**
www.aacn.org

American Association of Diabetes Educators
100 West Monroe Street, 4th Floor
Chicago, IL 60603-1901
(312) 424-2426 or 1-800-338-DMED

American Association of Neuroscience Nurses
224 North Des Plaines, Suite 601
Chicago, IL 60661
(312) 993-0043

American Association of Nurse Anesthetists
222 South Prospect Avenue
Park Ridge, IL 60068-4001
(847) 692-7050

American Association of Occupational Health Nurses
50 Lenox Pointe
Atlanta, GA 30324
(404) 262-1162

American Association of Spinal Cord Injury Nurses
75-20 Astoria Boulevard
Jackson Heights, NY 11370-1177
(718) 803-3782

American Association of Nurse-Midwives
818 Connecticut Avenue NW, Suite 900
Washington, DC 20006
(202) 728-9860

American Nephrology Nurses' Association
East Holly Avenue, Box 56
Pitman, NJ 08071
(609) 256-2320

American Psychiatric Nurses' Association
1200 19th Street NW, Suite 300
Washington, DC 20036
(202) 857-1133

American Public Health Association/Public Health Nursing
1015 15th Street NW, 3rd Floor
Washington, DC 20005
(202) 789-5600

American Society of Ophthalmic Registered Nurses
Box 193030
San Francisco, CA 94119
(415) 561-8513

American Society of Post-Anesthesia Nurses
6900 Grove Road
Thorofare, NJ 08086
(609) 845-5557

**Association for Professionals in Infection Control and
   Epidemiology, Inc.**
1016 Sixteenth Street NW, 6th Floor
Washington, DC 20036
(202) 296-2742

Association of Operating Room Nurses
2170 South Parker Road, Suite 300
Denver, CO 80231-5711
(303) 755-6300

Association of Rehabilitation Nurses
4700 West Lake Avenue
Glenview, IL 60025-1485
(708) 966-3433

Association of Women's Health, Obstetric, and Neonatal Nurses
700 14th Street NW, Suite 600
Washington, DC 20005-2019
(202) 662-1608

Dermatology Nurses' Association
North Woodbury Road Box 56
Pitman, NJ 08071
(609) 256-2330

Emergency Nurses Association
219 Higgins Road
Park Ridge, IL 60068
(708) 698-9400

Intravenous Nurses Society
Fresh Pond Square
10 Fawcett Street
Cambridge, MA 02138
(617) 441-3008

American Association of Nurse Attorneys
720 Light Street
Baltimore, MD 21230
(410) 752-3318

American Holistic Nurses' Association
PO Box 2130
Flagstaff, AZ 86003
E-mail: **ANHA-Flag@flaglink.com**

American Organization of Nurse Executives
325 7th Street NW, Suite 700
Washington, DC 20004
(202) 626-2240

Association of Nurses in AIDS Care
11250 Roger Bacon Drive, Suite 8
Reston, VA 22091-5202
(703) 925-0081

Hospice Nurses Association
5512 North Umberland Street
Pittsburgh, PA 15217
(412) 687-3231

National Association of Neonatal Nurses
1304 Sandpoint Boulevard, Suite 280
Petaluma, CA 94954-6859
(707) 762-5588

National Association of Orthopaedic Nurses, Inc.
North Woodbury Road, Box 56
Pitman, NJ 08071
(609) 256-2310

National Association of Pediatric Nurse Associates and Practitioners
1101 Kings Highway North, Suite 206
Cherry Hill, NJ 08034
(609) 667-1773

National Association of School Nurses, Inc.
PO Box 1300
Lamplighter Lane
Scarborough, ME 04074-1300
(207) 883-2117

National Flight Nurses Association
216 Higgins Road
Park Ridge, IL 60068
(847) 698-1733

Oncology Nursing Society
501 Holiday Drive
Pittsburgh, PA 15220
(412) 921-7373

Sigma Theta Tau International, Honor Society of Nursing
550 West North
Indianapolis, IN 46202
(317) 634-8171
www.stti.iupui.edu

Respiratory Nursing Society
7794 Grow Drive
Pensacola, FL 32514-7072
(850) 474-8869

Society for Vascular Nursing
309 Winter Street
Norwood, MA 02062
(781) 762-3630

Other Titles in the
Majoring in Your Life Series

Majoring in the Rest of Your Life: Career Secrets for College Students by Carol Carter
Hardcover 0-374-19924-8 / $21.00
Paperback 0-374-52451-3 / $10.00
Series editor Carol Carter presents high school and college students with a practical strategy to get you from your first semester in freshman year to your first job. Chock-full of the kind of personal student experiences and advice that has become the hallmark of the *Majoring in Your Life* series, *Majoring in the Rest of Your Life* can help you discover what you enjoy doing and how to land the job of your dreams.

Majoring in Engineering: How to Get from Your Freshman Year to Your First Job by John Garcia
Hardcover 0-374-19919-1 / $21.00
Paperback 0-374-52441-6 / $10.00
Garcia introduces prospective engineers to the profession and shows them how to evaluate their talents for it; how to choose the right engineering school; how to decide on the right concentration (civil, mechanical, chemical, etc.); how to survive freshman physics and other such horrors; and, finally, how to get a job.

Majoring in Law: It's Not Right for Everyone. Is it Right for You? by Stefan Underhill
Paperback 0-374-52442-4 / $11.00
Underhill examines the good and not so good reasons why people become lawyers and, in the process, helps you determine whether it's the

best career for you. He describes the legal landscape, including private practice, public interest groups, and the government; shows how to make yourself more attractive to law schools and legal employers; and provides tips for surviving and distinguishing yourself in law school.